D1531898

Prayerfully Expecting

Other Books by the Author

Catholic Prayer Book for Mothers
The Heart of Motherhood

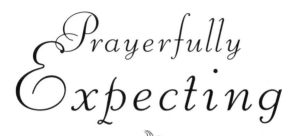

Prayerfully Expecting

A Nine-Month Novena
for Mothers to Be

DONNA-MARIE COOPER O'BOYLE

With illustrations by
CHALDEA EMERSON

A Crossroad Book
The Crossroad Publishing Company
New York

The Crossroad Publishing Company
831 Chestnut Ridge Road
Chestnut Ridge, NY 10977

www.crossroadpublishing.com

Printed in the United States of America on acid-free paper. The text of this book is set in 11/16 Goudy.

Library of Congress Cataloging-in-Publication Data

O'Boyle, Donna-Marie Cooper.

   Prayerfully expecting : a nine month novena for mothers
to be / Donna-Marie Cooper O'Boyle.
      p. cm.
   ISBN-13: 978-0-8245-2459-3 (alk. paper)
   ISBN-10: 0-8245-2459-4 (alk. paper)
1. Pregnant women – Prayer-books and devotions – English. 2. Pregnancy– Religious aspects – Christianity. 3. Mothers – Prayer-books and devotions–English. 4. Motherhood

Religious aspects –Christianity. 5. Novenas. I. Title.

BV4847.O255 2006

242'.6431–dc22

                                                          2006035301

2 3 4 5 6 7 8   A   16 15 14 13 12

With all of my heart to
all of my children:

Justin, Chaldea, Jessica, Joseph,
and Mary-Catherine.

I still remember vividly all of my pregnancies
with you, and I thank God for the
incredible gifts of all of you.

Contents

Apostolic Blessing from

Pope John Paul II

Shortly after the beatification of Blessed Teresa of Calcutta, Pope John Paul II imparted his apostolic blessing on Donna-Marie Cooper O'Boyle, her family, and her work *"as a pledge of joy and peace in our Lord Jesus Christ,"* and he promised his prayers and good wishes for Donna-Marie Cooper O'Boyle's work and writings on Mother Teresa of Calcutta.

(October 30, 2003)

Foreword by

Blessed Mother Teresa of Calcutta

Just as love begins at home, so also peace and the woman being the heart of the family — let us pray that we women realize the reason of existence is to love and be loved and through this love become an instrument of peace.

—Blessed Mother Teresa of Calcutta, October 26, 1991

Blessing by

Blessed Mother Teresa of Calcutta

Blessed Mother Teresa also said to the author of this book, "God has given you many gifts — make sure you use them for the glory of God and the good of the people. You will then make your life something beautiful for God. You have been created to be Holy. I assure you of my prayers and hope you pray for me also. Keep the joy of loving Jesus ever burning in your heart and share this joy with others." She continued, "My gratitude is my prayer for you that you may grow in the love of God through your beautiful thoughts of prayer you write and thus share with others.

"Your books on young mothers and expectant mothers are much needed. Yes, you may use some of the things I said on motherhood and family. I pray that God may bless your endeavors."

About this book, Blessed Mother Teresa said, "I pray that it does much good."

Foreword

Donna-Marie's book *Prayerfully Expecting* is a spiritual chalice of love, love for every human being, from the moment of conception, as unique, precious, and unrepeatable. Again and again, Donna-Marie affirms, as only a mother can, that motherhood is a commitment in faith, hope, and love; hence, the expectant mother literally makes a pilgrimage of prayer as she approaches the moment of childbirth. In this pilgrimage the mother walks with Mary, the Mother of Jesus, our Lord and Savior. The author structures the nine months of waiting for childbirth in the context of a novena, during which Saint Anne, Saint Joseph, and Saint Gerard Majella, the patron saint for expectant mothers, are also invoked. There is strong catechetical content to this novena; papal encyclicals such as *Humanae Vitae* are cited, along with some of the most memorable statements of Pope John Paul II. Various saints and theologians are quoted throughout. Alongside the devotional and the catechetical helps are pointed references to the child's development in the womb as the months of pregnancy progress. The way in which the author implements her idea of making a novena during the nine months before childbirth is especially relevant and beautiful.

Msgr. David Q. Liptak, DMin
Executive Editor of *The Catholic Transcript* and censor librorum for the Archdiocese of Hartford

Introduction

*But Jesus said, "Let the children come to me, and do not
hinder them; for to such belongs the kingdom of heaven."*
— MATTHEW 19:14, RSV (CE)

You have been blessed with the privilege of conceiving a
child, whose heart beats within you. Cradled inside you,
your unborn child will be nourished and kept warm in your
womb for the next nine months. What an incredible miracle!

Motherhood is truly a lofty and blessed vocation. By
responding to life with a generous "yes," you have entered into a
partnership with God, cooperating to bring a new soul into this
world. What could possibly be more worthwhile than this?

And isn't it fascinating that a pregnancy's duration is for
nine months? The perfect period of time for a novena of prayers
and reflection! Your pregnancy can become a distinctive inter-
lude of contemplation as you delight in your baby's movements
and life within you and prepare for his or her arrival. This reflective prayer journal was written to assist you in creating a prayerful, peaceful, and nurturing experience throughout your pregnancy to benefit you and your unborn baby.

By following and praying through this prayer book each month until your child's birth, your pregnancy will become a complete novena to Saint Anne — grandmother of Jesus, mother of our Blessed Mother, and the patron saint for mothers — and also a novena to Saint Gerard Majella, another saint for mothers. Additionally, you will pray the Rosary, meditating on the mysteries of Jesus's and Mary's lives as you reflect on your pregnancy. Many inspirational writings from the saints and our holy fathers are sprinkled throughout this book to help affirm a mother's dignity and worth. Each month as you continue on your pilgrimage during your pregnancy, you will also be kept informed about your baby's progress.

Don't hesitate to write on the pages of this book; your words will transform it into a wonderful journal to grow in faith with and to cherish in years to come when you reminisce on this special era of your life. Make it your own by writing your own prayer of blessing for your pregnancy in the front cover of the book. There is space throughout to write thoughts, prayers, and reflections. And there are blank pages where you can attach pictures of your family, of you as your belly grows, or even your ultrasound.

Relax and take your time each month as you go through the readings and reflections and as you pray. You may read through the chapter pertaining to your current month of pregnancy once or you may read parts of it several times during that particular month. You may also read a couple of readings, prayers, and reflections at various times throughout the month. You decide how you would like to use this prayer journal.

Try to put yourself in a spiritual and prayerful frame of mind each time you pick up this journal. You may want to ask our Lord to enlighten your mind and strengthen you both physically and spiritually during this novena of preparation for the birth of your child. Ask also for all of the graces possible to become the mother that you are destined to be. The quiet times that you experience during this pregnancy can be a retreat from the hectic pace of the world and a wonderful occasion of prayer and contemplation, enabling you to grow closer to God as your child grows within you.

By giving yourself the time to rest, reflect, and pray while you are carrying your precious child, you will most certainly provide a sense of peace and tranquility for both you and your baby, while being open to the many graces that our Heavenly Father has prepared for you!

Listen to the Lord's gentle promptings in your soul. Be at peace and enjoy this most beautiful time of your life when, because of God's grace and the love you share with your husband, you are carrying within you the most precious gift ever: a dear child of God. May God bless you and your unborn child in great abundance!

Women are builders of life and they know the qualities demanded of them and developed in them by the long period of gestation of children. They have a great capacity to love the child, which is to be born and to live by that hope, in spite of delay, problems, trials.

Women are capable of giving themselves without counting the cost "in order that human beings may have life" — all and especially that of the soul, through grace, that they may have it in abundance, that is to say, in the fullness of the Gospel, the sacraments and the Church.

Their devotion is often more intuitive than that of men. They are better able to discern the aspirations, the distresses, even unacknowledged, of humanity and to sense what is the appropriate response. Such intuition leads spontaneously to concrete initiatives: "It is man's nature to have ideas; it is woman's to act." But one should not force this antithesis.

In her work, it is easier for a woman to maintain continuity and faithfulness to life as it unfolds. Her faith in life sustains her faith in grace and gives her the patience needed for the work of natural and supernatural education.

— DANS LE CADRE, July 1976

Your First Month

As for Mary, she treasured all these things and pondered them in her heart.

— LUKE 2:19, NJB

Human life is sacred —from its very inception it reveals the creating hand of God.

—POPE JOHN XXIII, Mater et Magistra

WHAT'S HAPPENING WITH YOUR BABY?

*D*uring the first month in the womb, your baby, which is an embryo at this point, will increase in size about ten thousand times and increase in weight almost three thousand times.

Your child will actually transform from a single cell into an embryo with a head, a trunk, and the rudiments of organs. By the end of the first month, the embryo, once an unformed microscopic unit of protoplasm, will comprise millions of intricately organized groups of cells, which have specific functions. Your baby will become approximately one-fourth to one-half of an inch long from its head to its heel.

By the end of this first month, your baby will have completed the greatest size increase and physical change of a lifetime. Take good care of yourself now and throughout your pregnancy. Your little one depends on you for his or her very existence.

* * *

Take a few moments to fill in the information below (before you forget!).

Date of conception (not always known): _____

Estimated due date: _____

Date I found out about my pregnancy: _____

Where I was when I found out about my pregnancy: _____

_____

_____

_____

How I knew I was pregnant: _____

_____

_____

_____

How I shared the wonderful news with the new father: _____

_____

_____

_____

His reactions and responses: _____

_____

_____

_____

How I told my family the wonderful news: _____

_____

_____

_____

Their reactions and responses: _____

_____

_____

_____

What it means to me to be chosen by God to carry the gift of this precious child within my womb: _____

_____

_____

_____

_____

_____

_____

_____

_____

_____

_____

_____

_____

_____

*M*otherhood involves a special communion with the mystery of life, as it develops in the mother's womb. The mother is filled with wonder at this mystery of life, and understands with unique intuition what is happening inside her. In the light of the beginning the mother accepts and loves as a person the child she is carrying in her womb. This unique contact with the new human being developing within her gives rise to an attitude towards human beings — not only towards her own child, but every human being — which profoundly marks the woman's personality. It is commonly thought that women are more capable than men of paying attention to another person, and that motherhood develops this predisposition even more.

— POPE JOHN PAUL II, *Mulieri s Dignitatem*

THANK YOU, LORD, FOR
ENTRUSTING ME WITH THIS CHILD

Thank you, dear Lord, for entrusting me with a special communion with the mystery of life as it blossoms within my being. You have given me the gift of a child, who is growing in my womb, being nurtured by my life and love. This reality would be almost too intense for me to fathom, but your grace and love gives me a motherly intuition that allows me to understand the meaning and beauty of life as it actually has been created within me. Please keep me safe, Lord, and watch over me and my unborn child. Help me to mother my unborn child with love and care as my commitment and dedication to him or her deepen each day. Please grant me all of the graces I need to be the mother I am destined to be. Thank you, Lord, for this precious gift of life! Amen.

Time to Reflect

Take some time to reflect on the role of motherhood and also on the love you have for your unborn child. During your reflective times, quiet times, and even during your busy times, lift your heart to the Lord in prayer. Blessed Teresa of Calcutta spoke about the need to pray when she said, "Try to feel the need for prayer often during the day and take the trouble to pray. Prayer makes the heart large enough until it can contain God's gift of Himself. Ask and seek, and your heart will grow big enough to receive Him and keep Him as your own."

When expecting, learn to seek our Lord often as you go through your days caring for your unborn baby and your household. You can start each day with an offering of your heart to our

Lord. Ask him to bless your day and offer him all your prayers, works, joys, and sufferings of the day. As you go about your routine and at quiet times, lift your heart to our Lord, thanking him for his love, asking for his graces, and asking him to increase your faith. Strive to retreat within your heart as often as you can throughout your pregnancy, asking our Lord for all that you need to become the mother you were meant to be.

PRAYER TO THE HOLY FAMILY

Lord Jesus Christ, you were raised by Mary and Joseph within the Holy Family in Nazareth. Your home was humble and holy. Help us discover the holiness in simplicity and obedience to our state of life. Help us to imitate the virtues of the Holy Family as we remain faithful to our daily duties. Please also help us to find ways to seek out solitude even in the midst of our busy lives so that we may unite our hearts with yours, dear Jesus. Please, Blessed Mother Mary and good Saint Joseph, pray for us and protect us. Amen.

ACT OF FAITH

I firmly believe in You, my God, with all of my heart and that You are one God in three divine persons, Father, Son, and Holy Spirit. I believe that Your Divine Son, Jesus, died for all of mankind, suffering for our sins, and I believe that he will come again to judge the living and the dead. I believe these and all the truths that our Catholic Church teaches. Thank you for the gift of faith. Please increase it in my heart. Amen.

ccording to the plan of God, marriage is the foundation of the wider community of the family, since the very institution of marriage and conjugal love are ordained to the procreation and education of children, in whom they find their crowning.

In its most profound reality, love is essentially a gift; and conjugal love, while leading the spouses to the reciprocal knowledge which makes them one flesh, does not end with the couple, because it makes them capable of the greatest possible gift, the gift by which they become cooperators with God for giving life to a new human person. Thus the couple, while giving themselves to one another, give not just themselves but also the reality of children who are a living reflection of their love, a permanent sign of conjugal unity and a living and inseparable synthesis of their being a father and a mother.

When they become parents, spouses receive from God the gift of a new responsibility. Their parental love is called to become for the children the visible sign of the very love of God, from whom every family in heaven and on earth is named.

— POPE JOHN PAUL II, *Familiaris Consortio*

REMEMBERING THE ANNUNCIATION

Just as Mary, our Blessed Mother, responded with faith and trust and great humility when the Angel of the Lord appeared to her, so a mother also says, "Be it done unto me according to thy word," when she accepts the gift of a new life within her.

MOTHER'S DAILY PRAYER
FOR HER CHILDREN

O Mary, Immaculate Virgin, Mother of our Lord Jesus Christ, patroness of all mothers, I commend my beloved children to the Most Sacred Heart of your son, Jesus, and to your Immaculate Heart. Please assist our family and keep us always in your care. Please protect us from the snares of the devil and keep us on the road that leads to life. Help me to realize my sublime mission as a mother and help me be faithful to my duties for the good of my family and the good of the entire family of God.

Most Sacred Heart of Jesus, have mercy on us.
Immaculate Heart of Mary, pray for us.
My Guardian Angel, pray for me.
Holy Guardian Angel of our family, pray for us.
Saint Michael, pray for us.
Saint Joseph, husband of Mary, pray for us.
Saint Anne, mother of Mary, pray for us.
Saint Elizabeth, pray for us.
Saint Elizabeth Ann Seton, pray for us.
Saint Monica, pray for us.

Saint Augustine, pray for us.
Saint Gerard Majella, pray for us.
Blessed Mother Teresa of Calcutta, pray for us. Amen.

THE MAGNIFICAT

My soul proclaims the greatness of the Lord
and my spirit rejoices in God my Saviour;
because he has looked upon the humiliation of his servant. Yes, from
now onwards all generations will call me blessed, for the Almighty
has done great things for me.
Holy is his name, and his faithful love extends age after age to those
who fear him.
He has used the power of his arm, he has routed the arrogant of heart.
He has pulled down princes from their thrones and raised high the lowly.
He has filled the starving with good things, sent the rich away empty.
He has come to the help of Israel his servant, mindful of his faithful
love—according to the promise he made to our ancestors— of his
mercy to Abraham and to his descendants for ever.

— LUKE 1:46–55, NJB

* * *

A thought, a prayer, a reflection...

Dear fathers and mothers believe in your vocation, that beautiful vocation of marriage and parenthood which God has given you. Believe that God is with you — for all parenthood in heaven and on earth takes its name from Him. Do not think that anything you will do in this life is more important than to be a good Christian father and mother.

— POPE JOHN PAUL II, October 1, 1979

Praying a Novena

A novena is a distinctive time for prayer. It usually lasts for a period of nine days and consists of public or private prayer for a special occasion or petition, sometimes invoking a particular saint for help. The practice of saying a novena originates with the nine days that the disciples and Mary spent together in passionate prayer between Ascension and Pentecost Sunday. Over the centuries the Catholic Church has indulged many novenas and many graces are said to be granted to the people praying the novenas. The number nine is significant when it comes to novenas and by praying through the novenas in this prayer book, you will transform your nine-month pregnancy into a beautiful novena of prayer, surely pleasing our Lord and you will receive graces for yourself, your unborn baby, and your family.

NOVENA TO
SAINT ANNE 1

Catholics have looked to Saint Anne, Jesus's grandmother, throughout history for her intercessory prayers. She was considered to be a valiant woman, strong in her faultless virtue, protecting her home, her husband's honor, her children's future. She kept her people's traditions and laws and opened her heart to God in all things.

PRAYER TO SAINT ANNE

Heavenly Father, I begin my novena prayers as I begin this pregnancy. I know that You chose Saint Anne and blessed her with the honor of being the grandmother of Your son, Jesus Christ. Please grant in Thy mercy that all who make this novena in her honor will be aided by her powerful intercession with You. I especially ask for Saint Anne's intercession for my pregnancy and specifically during this first month. I ask this through Jesus Christ, Your son, who lives and reigns with You in the unity of the Holy Spirit. Amen.

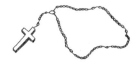

Praying the Rosary

The Rosary is a beautiful form of prayer and a fitting one to recite throughout a pregnancy. It has been the most popular and enduring of all Catholic devotions since the Middle Ages. Pope John Paul II said, "From my youthful years this prayer has held an important place in my spiritual life. The Rosary has accompanied me in moments of joy and in moments of difficulty. To it I have entrusted any number of concerns: in it I have always found comfort."

While meditating on the mysteries of the Rosary, an expectant mother will come closer to our Lord Jesus and his Blessed Mother and receive many graces, as well. This renowned prayer can be said at any time of the day or night, while traveling, at rest, at quiet times, and even during various activities such as taking a walk. Many people find that the repetitive prayers of the Hail Mary said while meditating on a particular mystery of the Rosary helps to calm them and helps them to focus their heart and mind, becoming more open to the Lord.

If you are without Rosary beads, you may substitute your ten fingers for the beads of a decade. There may be times when you cannot complete an entire Rosary. Praying the Rosary one decade at a time throughout the day is fine and pleasing to our Lord and his Blessed Mother. They know you may be tired during your pregnancy or may be busy looking after your other children and the household. Our Lord knows the busyness of your life. After all, don't forget — our Lord made you the mom!

THE JOYFUL MYSTERIES
OF THE ROSARY

I. THE ANNUNCIATION

The Angel Gabriel called to you: "Ave Maria." O Mary, Queen of Angels, you represented humanity, and the Angel Gabriel was God's messenger on that most joyful day that changed and renewed the face of the earth forever. You were asked to consent to Jesus's conception through the overshadowing of the Holy Spirit. You understood what God's miraculous grace for you would accomplish and replied, "Let it be done to me according to Thy word." Please intercede for me and my unborn baby, Blessed Mother, as I recite these beads of the holy Rosary in your honor.

Our Father, ten Hail Marys, Glory Be to the Father, Fatima Prayer — O my Jesus, forgive us our sins; save us from the fires of hell; lead all souls to Heaven, especially those most in need. Amen.

Our Lady of the Rosary, please obtain for me from your son the grace of humility so that I may recite the beads with devotion. Please watch over my unborn baby and me.

II. THE VISITATION

Dear Mary, your brave and selfless response upon hearing of your aged cousin Elizabeth's pregnancy should teach me about holy selflessness, which is a virtue necessary in my vocation of motherhood. You brought great joy to Elizabeth and her husband, Zachary, when you visited their home in Judea. Saint John the

Baptist leapt for joy in his mother's womb at the sound of your greeting because you were carrying holy baby Jesus inside you. You professed your vocation as God's mother when you replied to Elizabeth's greeting with the words of the Magnificat: "My soul magnifies the Lord and my spirit rejoices in God my Savior." Dear Mother Mary, please help me to see the sublimity in my own vocation as a mother carrying a child of God in my own womb.

Our Father, ten Hail Marys, Glory Be to the Father, Fatima Prayer — O my Jesus, forgive us our sins; save us from the fires of hell; lead all souls to Heaven, especially those most in need. Amen.

Our Lady of the Rosary, please obtain for me from your son the grace of fraternal charity so that I may give of myself to those in need, loving him or her by God's grace. Please watch over my unborn baby and me.

III. THE NATIVITY

Jesus, our Lord and king, was born into poverty, resting his sacred head on hay in an animal's manger. His mother, Mary, and step-father, Joseph, had been shunned from the inn and forced to find a place in which the Savior of the world could be born. This holy family was poor in spirit but rich in love and grace. Jesus, you did not want us to fear approaching you, who are full of power and glory, so you allowed yourself a simple life, beginning with your birth in a stable. Both the rich and poor come to you — Magi and shepherds. You welcome us all. Help me to run fearlessly into your arms.

Our Father, ten Hail Marys, Glory Be to the Father, Fatima Prayer — O my Jesus, forgive us our sins; save us from the fires of

hell; lead all souls to Heaven, especially those most in need. Amen.

Mary, Queen of the Rosary, please obtain for me from your son, the grace that I may be poor in spirit. Please watch over my unborn baby and me.

IV. PRESENTATION OF THE CHILD JESUS IN THE TEMPLE

Blessed Mother Mary, there was no need for purification or redemption of you or Jesus, yet you were obedient to the law of your people. Mosaic Law required a mother to stay home for seven days after the birth of a son and then an additional thirty-three days. Every first-born son had to be offered to the Lord and redeemed by a pair of turtledoves, or two young pigeons. You and your husband, Joseph, offered the turtledoves symbolizing immaculate purity, and innocence of Mother and Child. Jesus was Immaculate Purity and you were the Immaculate Conception. Your mother, Anne, blessed you, while Simeon prophesied that a sword of sorrow would pierce your soul because of your son, Jesus.

Our Father, ten Hail Marys, Glory Be to the Father, Fatima Prayer — O my Jesus, forgive us our sins; save us from the fires of hell; lead all souls to Heaven, especially those most in need. Amen.

Our Lady of the Rosary, please obtain for me from your son the grace of chastity in thought, word, and deed, so that I may avoid sins of the flesh. Please watch over my unborn baby and me.

V. FINDING THE CHILD JESUS IN THE TEMPLE

"Did you not know that I must be about my Father's business?" were the words your son replied to you, dear Blessed Mother, when you asked why he had left you and Joseph without telling you. Your motherly heart was heavy with concern about your lost twelve-year-old son, Jesus. Unbeknownst to you, he remained in Jerusalem when you and Joseph headed back to Nazareth. Jesus struck up an acquaintance with the doctors of the Law in the Temple, taking part in discussions. The doctors were amazed at your son's knowledge. You surely welcomed him with open arms when you found him in the Temple, proud that he was busy about his Father's business, at the same time relieved that he was safe.

Our Father, ten Hail Marys, Glory Be to the Father, Fatima Prayer — O my Jesus, forgive us our sins; save us from the fires of hell; lead all souls to Heaven, especially those most in need. Amen.

Our Lady of the Rosary, please obtain for me from your son the grace of zeal so that I may be industrious for the things of God. Please watch over my unborn baby and me.

Queen of the most holy Rosary, pray for us.

O Mary, conceived without sin, pray for us who have recourse to thee.

Pope John Paul II reflected on a mother's role in "On the Dignity and Vocation of Women" when he said, "Mary's words at the annunciation — 'let it be done to me according to your word' — signify the woman's readiness for the gift of self and her readiness to accept new life."

NOVENA TO
SAINT GERARD MAJELLA 1

Saint Gerard, expectant mothers and their families often invoke you. I confidently call upon you, imploring you to watch over me and my unborn baby during my pregnancy. Please intercede for me to the Blessed Trinity that my baby and I will remain well and that my baby may see his or her way to baptism. Please pray also that after having lived as good Christians here on earth, we may both one day be united in the everlasting happiness of Heaven. Amen.

Our Father, Hail Mary, Glory Be to the Father Saint Gerard, please pray for us.

PRAYER TO OUR BLESSED MOTHER

Dear Blessed Mother Mary, you who are the mother of all mothers, please guide me, protect me, and keep me always in your care. Help me to prepare for the birth of my baby by tending to my pregnancy with care. Please pray to your son, Jesus, for me, that he will grant me the graces I need to become a good and loving mother. Help me to learn by your example: your quiet, humble service, your loving obedience, your total self-giving, and your peaceful inner strength. Help me to offer my pregnancy to your son, giving him the sufferings as well as the joys, that God's holy will may be fulfilled in my life and in my family. Hail Mary, full of grace, the Lord is with thee, blessed are Thou amongst women, and blessed is the fruit of thy womb, Jesus. Holy Mary,

Mother of God, pray for us sinners, now and at the hour of our death. Amen.

PRAYER FOR A FAMILY

O dear Jesus, I confidently ask you to grant my family the graces that we need to serve you well. Please, dear Lord, protect and bless all of us who are present or away, living and deceased. Help us to hold tight to each other and know that prayer will unite our hearts and souls and keep us together in your love. Amen.

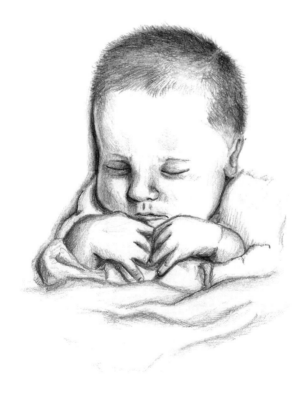

A GRACE-FILLED MONTH

You have completed the first month of your pregnancy — the first month of your new child's life within you. Your unborn baby has grown in leaps and bounds, seemingly silently within your womb, almost secretly living and thriving hidden inside you — a precious blessing of new life that God has bestowed on you.

A month of preparation for motherhood has passed, a month of prayer and reflection. Hopefully you have taken time out this month to pray and seek solitude in which to grow in holiness. Thank our dear Lord for this new life that has begun inside you, for this opportunity to house and nurture one of God's children.

PRAYER FROM MY HEART

A prayer to my Lord from my heart in thanksgiving for this most beautiful gift of new life within me:

Oh dear Lord

* * *

Reflections on My First Month of Pregnancy

_____

_____

_____

_____

_____

_____

_____

_____

_____

_____

_____

_____

_____

_____

_____

_____

_____

_____

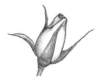

Your Second Month

In truth I tell you, anyone who does not welcome the Kingdom of God like a little child will never enter it.

— LUKE 18:17, NJB

The future of humanity passes by way of the family. It is therefore indispensable and urgent that every person of good will should endeavor to save and foster the values and requirements of the family.

— POPE JOHN PAUL II, *Familiaris Consortio*

WHAT'S HAPPENING WITH YOUR BABY?

*D*uring this second month of life, your child's earliest reflexes begin. In the first three weeks of the second month, the seemingly primitive embryo becomes a well-proportioned, small-scale baby. Your baby's neural tube (which will become your baby's brain and spinal cord), heart, digestive tract, sensory organs, and arm and leg buds will begin to form. By the seventh week its face is formed, with eyes, ears, nose, lips, tongue, and even milk teeth buds in the gums. Your baby's small arms will develop hands, with fingers and thumbs. The legs will grow a little slower, as knees, ankles, and toes become recognizable.

Your baby's brain already sends out impulses that coordinate the functioning of other organs. Your baby's heart beats sturdily. During this period of rapid cell growth, the new cells are especially susceptible to physical and chemical influences, good or bad. That is why you should not take any medications now or at any time during your pregnancy without your doctor's consent and supervision. Also, you should refrain from using tobacco, alcohol, or drugs because of their adverse effects on yourself and your unborn baby.

At two months in the uterus, your baby's palm prints and footprints already have permanently engraved lines on the skin. By the sixth week, a complete skeleton will have formed, although it is not yet made of bone, still cartilage.

Although we know that your baby's life began at conception, by the end of the second month, an embryologist will now call the embryo (from the Greek, to swell, to teem within) a fetus (from the Latin, young one or offspring) because of the baby's features, which are now clearly evident.

Although both together are parents of their child, the woman's motherhood constitute a special part in this shared parenthood, and the most demanding part. Parenthood — even though it belongs to both — is realized more fully in the woman, especially in the prenatal period. It is the woman who pays directly for this shared generation, which literally absorbs the energies of her body and soul. It is therefore necessary that the man be fully aware that in their shared parenthood he owes a special debt to the woman. No program of "equal rights" between women and men is valid unless it takes this fact fully into account.

— POPE JOHN PAUL II, *Mulieris Dignitatem*

PRAYER TO THE HOLY FAMILY

Humbly hidden with his family, our Lord Jesus spent his first thirty years quietly with his mother, Mary, and his foster father, Joseph. Please, Lord Jesus, help me to meditate upon the mysteries of the Holy Family and strive to imitate their virtues as I live out my role in the vocation of motherhood. Amen.

ACT OF HOPE

O dear God, I hope to obtain pardon for my sins, trusting in your almighty and infinite mercy. I pray for your grace, asking through Jesus Christ, my Lord and Redeemer. My hope will remain in the Lord. Amen.

Lo, sons are a heritage from the Lord,
the fruit of the womb a reward.
Like arrows in the hand of a warrior
are the sons of one's youth. Happy is the man who has his quiver
    full of them!
He shall not be put to shame
when he speaks with his enemies at the gate.

— Psalm 127:3–5, RSV (CE)

MOTHER'S DAILY PRAYER
FOR HER CHILDREN

O Mary, Immaculate Virgin, Mother of our Lord Jesus Christ, patroness of all mothers, I commend my beloved children to the Most Sacred Heart of your son, Jesus, and to your Immaculate Heart. Please assist our family and keep us always in your care. Please protect us from the snares of the devil and keep us on the road that leads to life. Help me to realize my sublime mission as a mother and help me be faithful to my duties for the good of my family and the good of the entire family of God.

Most Sacred Heart of Jesus, have mercy on us.

Immaculate Heart of Mary, pray for us.

My Guardian Angel, pray for me.
Holy Guardian Angel of our family, pray for us.
Saint Michael, pray for us.
Saint Joseph, husband of Mary, pray for us.
Saint Anne, mother of Mary, pray for us.
Saint Elizabeth, pray for us.
Saint Elizabeth Ann Seton, pray for us.
Saint Monica, pray for us.
Saint Augustine, pray for us.
Saint Gerard Majella, pray for us.
Blessed Mother Teresa of Calcutta, pray for us.
Amen.

WOMAN'S DOUBLE DESTINY

Pope Pius XII described the sublimity in a mother's mission as a profound weaving together of her physical structure and her spirituality, her tender thoughts and her loving heart. He told us of a woman's double destiny, which begins with her acceptance of her motherly role. He said, "There can be no doubt that the primary function and sublime mission of woman is motherhood, and, in accordance with the lofty goal which the Creator Himself has set in the order He has chosen, this dominates the life of woman intensively and extensively. Her very physical structure, her spiritual qualities, the richness of her sentiments, combine to make woman a mother, to such an extent that motherhood represents the ordinary way for woman to reach her true perfection (even in the moral order) and, at the same time, to achieve her double destiny — that on earth and that in heaven.

Motherhood is not the ultimate foundation of woman's dignity but it does give her such splendor and so great a role in the working out of human destiny that this by itself is enough to make every man on the face of the earth, great or small as he may be, bow with reverence and love in the presence of his own mother" (October 14, 1956).

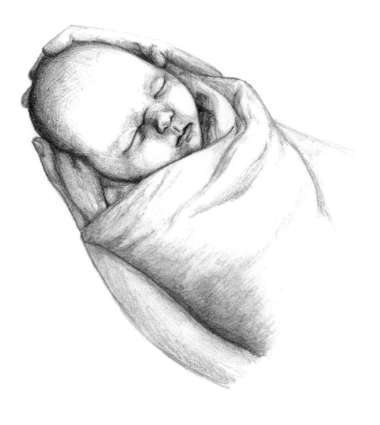

hat was the Good News that Christ had come to give? That God is love. That God loves you. God loves me. That God has made you and made me for better things to love and to be loved. We are not just a number in the world. That's why it is so wonderful to recognize the presence of that unborn child, the gift of God. The greatest gift of God to a family is the child, because it is the fruit of love.

And it is so wonderful to think that God has created a child, has created you, has created me, that very poor person in the street. The hungry person, that naked person, He has created in His image, to love and be loved, not to be just a number.

And we read something very beautiful in the Scripture, also, where God speaks, and He says: "Even if a mother could forget her child, I will not forget you. I have carved you in the palm of My hand. You are precious to me. I have called you by name."

That is why as soon as a child is born, we give it a name, the name God has called from all eternity — to love and be loved.

— BLESSED TERESA OF CALCUTTA

NOVENA TO
SAINT ANNE 2

Blessed Mother Mary grew up in the peaceful loving home of her parents, Joachim and Anne. Mary learned from her mother Anne's blessed example. Mary surely earned the lessons of a wife's devotion and diligence and a mother's peaceful loving heart.

Mary watched her mother's devotion and received the benefits of it in her home. She surely saw her mother's dedication and great tenderness and love, which Anne put into her motherly tasks. Mary began to understand the mystery of the power in doing small things with great love — of giving oneself in service to the family in obedience to one's state in life.

PRAYER TO SAINT ANNE

Dear Saint Anne, patroness of mothers, please listen to my humble prayers to you. I ask you to continue to guide me throughout this month when my baby is growing within me. Pray to the Heavenly Father, please, to grant me the graces I most need so that I will mother my child with a pure love and all the devotion of my heart. Guide me, please, to look for quiet moments to seek our Lord so that I will use this pregnancy wisely to be open to God's love for me and my baby in a special way. Help me to come closer to your daughter, Mary, as I pray throughout this pregnancy. Amen.

PRAYER TO JESUS

Dear Jesus, here I am in the first trimester of my pregnancy, seeking your love, grace, and guidance. Be with me, Lord, as I go through these days of my second month. Help me to choose quiet times to rest, relax, and pray. Show me your love, and help me open my heart more fully to you. Amen.

May mothers, young women and girls not listen to those who tell them that working at a secular job, succeeding in a secular profession, is more important than the vocation of giving life and caring for this life as a mother.

— POPE JOHN PAUL II, October 1, 1979

HUMAN LIFE IS SACRED

Human life is sacred and inviolable at every moment of existence, including the initial phase which precedes birth. All human beings, from their mother's womb, belong to God who searches them and knows them, who forms them and knits them together with his own hands, who gazes on them when they are tiny shapeless embryos and already sees in them the adults of tomorrow whose days are numbered and whose vocation is even now written in the "book of life" (cf. Ps 139:1, 13–16). There too, when they are still in their mother's womb — as many passages of the Bible bear witness — they are the personal objects of God's loving and fatherly providence.

— POPE JOHN PAUL II, *Evangelium Vitae*

DEAR MARY

Dear Mary, please remind me that my heart is firmly set on the goal of providing a nurturing home in my womb and in my household for my baby. Keep me close to you and your son, Jesus, so that I may seek Heaven above all else in this life. Help me to prepare my home for a new person. Show me how I encounter God within my family where we live in His peace in the blessedness of our daily life together. Amen.

THE SORROWFUL MYSTERIES
OF THE ROSARY

I. THE AGONY IN THE GARDEN

O dear Mary, Mother of Sorrows, you watched as your son, Jesus, was abandoned by his own friends and apostles. His disciples — Peter, James, and John — fell asleep in the garden and could not stay awake for even one hour with Jesus, leaving him alone to suffer his agony in the garden. Sweating blood and praying to the Father in Heaven, Jesus asked if the chalice of suffering could pass but truly wanted only the will of his Father, no matter what the cost. Please pray for me, Mary, that I will not fall asleep when your son, Jesus, is counting on me. And when I do, please remind me that I need only to ask for forgiveness and start again.

Our Father, ten Hail Marys, Glory Be to the Father, Fatima Prayer — O my Jesus, forgive us our sins; save us from the fires of hell; lead all souls to Heaven, especially those most in need. Amen.

Our Lady of the Rosary, please obtain for me from your son the grace of contrition and a pure heart so that I may be sorry for my sins, which caused Jesus to suffer. Please watch over my unborn baby and me.

II. THE SCOURGING AT THE PILLAR

O dear Mary, Mother of Sorrows, your heart must have been near breaking as you watched your son, Jesus, endure much suffering at the hands of the Roman soldiers. The lead balls at the ends of their whips tore through Jesus's skin, causing him to bleed. He was beaten inhumanly to almost unconsciousness, all while they mocked him and spat upon him.

Our Father, ten Hail Marys, Glory Be to the Father, Fatima Prayer — O my Jesus, forgive us our sins; save us from the fires of hell; lead all souls to Heaven, especially those most in need. Amen.

Our Lady of the Rosary, please obtain for me from your son the grace of patient endurance through the difficulties and sufferings in my life. Please watch over my unborn baby and me.

III. THE CROWNING WITH THORNS

O dear Mary, Mother of Sorrows, your son was mocked and ridiculed while a crown of thorns was pressed into his sacred head. This was the price he paid for love. They wrapped a purple robe around him and placed a reed in his hand to represent a scepter. They laughed in his face; they blasphemed him and bowed down before him in disrespect. Jesus did not strike back or talk back, but instead prayed to his Father in Heaven. Dear Mary, please remind me that as a Christian mother I may need to endure a bit of ridicule or mockery from others. Please remind me to pray and offer it to God rather than striking back.

Our Father, ten Hail Marys, Glory Be to the Father, Fatima Prayer — O my Jesus, forgive us our sins; save us from the fires of hell; lead all souls to Heaven, especially those most in need. Amen.

Our Lady of the Rosary, please obtain for me from your son the graces to be able to see suffering as a gift and an opportunity for conversion of hearts for myself and others when I offer it all to the Lord. Please watch over my unborn baby and me.

IV. THE CARRYING OF THE CROSS

O dear Mary, Mother of Sorrows, your son was already covered in wounds, and now he had a heavy wooden cross thrust upon his back and shoulders. While he struggled along carrying his Cross, Simon of Cyrene was forced to help carry the Cross so that Jesus could make it to Calvary. You were there, Mary, and your eyes met your son's eyes full of pain. Veronica mercifully wiped Jesus's face, and Jesus consoled the holy women. Dear Mary, help me to willingly carry my crosses with patience and love. Please ask our Lord for the graces I need to be like Veronica in my dealings with my family members and with others so that I may be a source of holy consolation.

Our Father, ten Hail Marys, Glory Be to the Father, Fatima Prayer — O my Jesus, forgive us our sins; save us from the fires of hell; lead all souls to Heaven, especially those most in need. Amen.

Our Lady of the Rosary, please obtain for me from your son the graces to understand the meaning in suffering and the strength to carry my crosses with love. Please watch over my unborn baby and me.

V. THE CRUCIFIXION

O dear Mary, Mother of Sorrows, your heart was breaking as you helplessly stood at the foot of the Cross. As he hung there, your son prayed for forgiveness from his Father for all that his enemies had done. He also promised Paradise to the good thief and entrusted John and you to each other. Your son cried out in thirst and commended his spirit to his Heavenly Father. Without heavenly assistance, you would have died right there with your son. Please, dear Mary, pray for me and my family that we will have the grace of perseverance in prayer throughout our lives so that we may come face to face with you in Heaven one day.

Our Father, ten Hail Marys, Glory Be to the Father, Fatima Prayer — O my Jesus, forgive us our sins; save us from the fires of hell; lead all souls to Heaven, especially those most in need. Amen.

Our Lady of the Rosary, please obtain for me from your son the grace to be obedient to my state in life and in all that is according to God's holy will. Please watch over my unborn child and me.

DEAR MARY

Queen of the most holy Rosary, pray for us.

O Mary, conceived without sin, pray for us who have recourse to thee.

UNDERSTANDING LOVE

You and I, being women, we have this tremendous thing in us, understanding love. I see that so beautifully in our people, in our poor women, who day after day, and everyday, meet suffering, accept suffering for the sake of their children. I have seen parents, mothers going without so many things, even resorting to begging, so that their children have what they need.

— BLESSED TERESA OF CALCUTTA

* * *

A thought, a prayer, a reflection...

$\mathcal{T}$he moral and spiritual strength of a woman is joined to her awareness that God entrusts the human being to her in a special way. Of course, God entrusts every human being to each and every other human being. But this entrusting concerns women in a special way — precisely by reason of their femininity — and this in particular determines their vocation.

The moral force of women, which draws strength from this awareness and this entrusting, expresses itself in a great number of figures of the Old Testament, of the time of Christ, and of later ages right up to our own day.

A woman is strong because of her awareness of this entrusting. Strong because of the fact that God "entrusts the human being to her" always and in every way, even in the situations of social discrimination in which she may find herself. This awareness and this fundamental vocation speak to women of the dignity, which they receive from God Himself, and this makes them "strong" and strengthens their vocation. Thus, the "perfect woman" (cf. Prov. 31:10) becomes an irreplaceable support and source of spiritual strength for other people, who perceive the great energies of her spirit. These "perfect women" are owed much by their families, and sometimes by whole nations.

— POPE JOHN PAUL II, *Mulieri s Dignitatem*

NOVENA TO
SAINT GERARD MAJELLA 2

O Saint Gerard, you trusted in God's divine providence in your life and made Him the center of your life. Please pray for me to do the same and put aside my worries or fears, trusting in God instead. Saint Gerard, expectant mothers and their families often invoke you. I confidently call upon you, imploring you to watch over me and my unborn baby during my pregnancy. I ask that you pray for special graces for me and for all expectant mothers. Please intercede for me to the Blessed Trinity that my baby and I will remain well and that my baby may see his or her way to baptism. Please pray also that after having lived as good Christians here on earth, we may both one day be united in the everlasting happiness of Heaven. Amen.

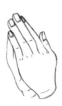

PRAYER TO OUR BLESSED MOTHER

Dear Mary, Mother of Jesus and my mother, please always be near me, be my guide and protector. Help me to learn from you and to imitate your virtues. Protect me, please, during this pregnancy. Help me to realize the great gift of new life within me that I have been entrusted with. Help me to care for myself properly and to be at peace so that my baby will begin it's new life in a safe and loving environment. Thank you, dear Blessed Mother Mary, for your beautiful love that you have for me. Thank you for the example that you set. Hail Mary, full of grace, the lord is with thee, blessed art thou amongst women and blessed is the fruit of thy womb, Jesus. Holy Mary, Mother of God, pray for us sinners, now and at the hour of our death. Amen.

PRAYER FOR A FAMILY

O dear Jesus, I confidently ask you to grant my family the graces that we need to serve you well. Please, dear Lord, protect and bless all of us who are present or away, living and deceased. Help us to hold tight to each other and know that prayer will unite our hearts and souls and keep us together in your love. Amen.

Our Father, Hail Mary, Glory Be, Saint Gerard, please pray for us. To ecstasy, I prefer the monotony of sacrifice.

— SAINT THÉRÈSE OF LISIEUX

A BLESSED MONTH

Your second month of pregnancy has come to a close. The weeks seemed to have flown by. Day by day, you approach your little one's birth. Hopefully, you haven't had much or any discomfort. Perhaps you have had some time to look forward with your husband to the joys that await the two of you in the very near future as you begin to get things ready, planning your lives, making room for a new little person. And as you progress through your pregnancy, you can relish the fact that your baby is thriving happily inside you — a cherished thought.

Thank our dear Lord for his great love for you, your husband, and your unborn child.

PRAYER FROM MY HEART

A prayer to my Lord from my heart in thanksgiving for this most beautiful gift of new life within me:

Oh dear Lord _____

_____

_____

_____

_____

_____

* * *

Reflections on My Second Month of Pregnancy

2

Your Third Month

Let the children come to me, do not stop them; for it is to such as these that the kingdom of God belongs.

— MARK 10:14, NJB

Motherhood is the fruit of the marriage union of a man and woman, of the biblical "knowledge" which corresponds to the "union of the two in one flesh" (cf. Gen 2:24). This brings about — on the woman's part — a special "gift of self," as an expression of that spousal love whereby the two are united to each other so closely that they become "one flesh." Biblical "knowledge" is achieved in accordance with the truth of the person only when the mutual self-giving is not distorted either by the desire of the man to become the "master" of his wife ("he shall rule over you") or by the woman remaining closed within her own instincts ("your desire shall be for your husband," Gen 3:16).

— POPE JOHN PAUL II, *Mulieris Dignitatem*

WHAT'S HAPPENING WITH
YOUR BABY?

*I*n your third month of pregnancy, your baby begins to be quite active, although still very small and weighing a little less than one ounce. At this point, when the brain signals, the muscles will respond with a kick or a turn. However, you will not be able to feel your lively baby moving around because of his or her tiny size and the fact that the newly formed muscles are weak. The cartilage is now becoming bone, and your baby is becoming more solid. More organs are developing; circulatory and urinary systems are operating. The distinctive differences between a girl and a boy are now apparent but a bit difficult to distinguish externally.

Your baby is now approximately three inches long, having gone through his or her most rapid development since conception. All this growth sometimes quietly takes place without the mother even knowing she is pregnant.

During the third month, a heartbeat can be heard with a stethoscope, and your baby's cute little face can now be seen on an ultrasound, squinting or frowning. He or she can now purse his or her lips and open his or her mouth.

Anticipating birth, your baby is already constantly rehearsing and improving the vital functions of breathing, eating, and motion. Because the actual structure of the muscles varies from child to child, your baby will show a distinct individuality in his or her behavior by the end of this third month.

PRAYER TO THE HOLY FAMILY

Lord Jesus Christ, you were raised by Mary and Joseph within the Holy Family in Nazareth. Your home was humble and holy. Help us discover the holiness in simplicity and obedience to our state of life. Help us to imitate the virtues of the Holy Family as we faithfully fulfill our daily duties. Please also help us to find ways to seek out solitude even in the midst of our busy lives so that we may unite our hearts with yours, dear Jesus. Please, Blessed Mother Mary and good Saint Joseph, pray for us and protect us. Amen.

ACT OF LOVE

O my God, You are all good and deserving of all my love. Therefore I love You, my Lord above all things. I pray to love my neighbors as myself for the love of You. I ask forgiveness for all of my sins and the grace to always forgive others. Amen.

MOTHER'S DAILY PRAYER
FOR HER CHILDREN

O Mary, Immaculate Virgin, Mother of our Lord Jesus Christ, patroness of all mothers, I commend my beloved children to the Most Sacred Heart of your son, Jesus, and to your Immaculate Heart. Please assist our family and keep us always in your care. Please protect us from the snares of the devil and keep us on the road that leads to life. Help me to realize my sublime mission as a mother and help me be faithful to my duties for the good of my family and the good of the entire family of God.

Most Sacred Heart of Jesus, have mercy on us.
Immaculate Heart of Mary, pray for us.
My Guardian Angel, pray for me.
Holy Guardian Angel of our family, pray for us.
Saint Michael, pray for us.
Saint Joseph, husband of Mary, pray for us.
Saint Anne, mother of Mary, pray for us.
Saint Elizabeth, pray for us.
Saint Elizabeth Ann Seton, pray for us.
Saint Monica, pray for us.
Saint Augustine, pray for us.
Saint Gerard Majella, pray for us.
Blessed Mother Teresa of Calcutta, pray for us. Amen.

PRAYER TO JESUS

O dear Jesus, you have put me here in the midst of my family, anticipating the birth of my child in a few short months. Help me to love my vocation of motherhood and my state in life. Help me to love my home as I get it ready for a blessed baby. Help me to realize that my home is my sanctuary, which, with love and devotion, I can convert to a cenacle of prayer. I need to be strong and to protect my family from the scandals and dangers of the world. Help me to look upon my home as another Nazareth, delighting in the solitude that it can bring my family, sheltered in the love within these walls. You show me that I have the power in my role as mother to transform our abode into an oasis of refreshment where my family can retreat from the world as we grow together daily in the blessed union of the family.

Help me to focus on my family, putting them first before attempting to accomplish anything outside the doors of my home. Being the heart of the home, I can be a much-needed instrument of peace. Amen.

NOVENA TO SAINT ANNE 3

Saint Anne and her husband, Joachim, beseeched God for a child and asked for only His holy will. The people of their day were unhappy and dreaming of the promised Savior. Saint Anne surely never dreamed that she would be given the privilege of being the grandmother of the Messiah. She never gave up hope that God would grant her a child, and in her old age, beautiful Mary was born to Anne and Joachim.

PRAYER TO SAINT ANNE

Dear Saint Anne, patroness of mothers, please listen to my humble prayers to you. I ask you to continue to guide me throughout this month when my baby is growing within me. Pray to the Heavenly Father, please, to grant me the graces I most need so that I will mother my child with a pure love and all of the devotion of my heart. Help me to always hold onto hope as you have done. Guide me, please, to look for quiet moments to seek our

Lord so that I will use this pregnancy wisely to be open to God's love for me and my baby in a special way. Help me to come closer to your daughter, Mary, as I pray throughout this pregnancy. Amen.

The motherhood of every woman, understood in the light of the Gospel, is similarly not only "of flesh and blood:" it expresses a profound "listening to the word of the living God" and a readiness to "safeguard" this Word, which is "the word of eternal life" (cf. John 6:68). For it is precisely those born of earthly mothers, the sons and daughters of the human race, who receive from the Son of God the power to become "children of God" (John 1:12). A dimension of the New Covenant in Christ's blood enters into human parenthood, making it a reality and a task for new creatures" (cf. 2 Cor. 5:17). The history of every human being passes through the threshold of a woman's motherhood; crossing it conditions "the revelation of the children of God" (cf. Rom. 8:19).

— POPE JOHN PAUL II, *Mulieri s Dignitatem*

Train up a child in the way he should go, and when he is old he will not depart from it.

— Proverbs 22:6, RSV (CE)

*T*he sanctuary in which every living person grows,
woman has a more alert sense and a more profound respect for the individual person and for his characteristics. She is a better judge of character. More easily than
a man, she is able to bring to flower the seeds of goodness,
which lie hidden in every soul.

— DANS LE CADRE, July 1976

THE GLORIOUS MYSTERIES
OF THE ROSARY

I. THE RESURRECTION

Dear Mother Mary, words could not possibly express the deep joy you must have felt on that Easter Sunday when your Son, Jesus, had risen from the tomb.

Our Father, ten Hail Marys, Glory Be to the Father, Fatima Prayer — O my Jesus, forgive us our sins; save us from the fires of hell; lead all souls to Heaven, especially those most in need. Amen.

Our Lady of the Rosary, please obtain for me from your son the grace of fervor in my prayers and a deep longing for things of God. Please watch over my unborn baby and me. Amen.

II. THE ASCENSION

Dear Mother Mary, the forty days following your son's resurrection were glorious. Jesus made Peter his Vicar on earth, head of the Church. He invested the apostles with his power and instructed them to "Go into all the world and preach the Gospel to the whole creation. He who believes and is baptized will be saved; but he who does not believe will be condemned" (Mark 16:15–16 [RSV]). Because his mission had been completed on earth, he led them to the top of Mount Olivet and blessed them before ascending to his Heavenly Father.

Our Father, ten Hail Marys, Glory Be to the Father, Fatima Prayer — O my Jesus, forgive us our sins; save us from the fires of

hell; lead all souls to Heaven, especially those most in need. Amen.

Our Lady of the Rosary, please obtain for me from your son the grace to see that just as the apostles were to preach the Gospel to every creature to the ends of the earth, I too am called to preach the Gospel, to live the Gospel in my family so that they will come close to Jesus and you and go out themselves to preach the Gospel so that all may reach Heaven one day. Please watch over my unborn baby and me. Amen.

III. THE DESCENT OF THE HOLY SPIRIT

Dear Mother Mary, Jesus fulfilled his promise to send the Holy Spirit to teach and comfort, when ten days after the Ascension, the mighty wind arose while you and the apostles were gathered together in the cenacle praying. Tongues of fire appeared over the heads of each apostle. The symbols of grace and holiness in the wind and fire initiated the Church's visible mission. The apostles would then go out to all nations with the Holy Spirit to preach the Good News.

Our Father, ten Hail Marys, Glory Be to the Father, Fatima Prayer — O my Jesus, forgive us our sins; save us from the fires of hell; lead all souls to Heaven, especially those most in need. Amen.

Our Lady of the Rosary, please obtain for me from your son the graces I need to be open to the Holy Spirit in my life. Pray for me please that I will strive to teach my child to be prayerful and open to the Holy Spirit. Please watch over my unborn baby and me. Amen.

IV. THE ASSUMPTION

Dear Mother Mary, you are the Queen of the Universe. You must have wanted to join your son, Jesus, in Heaven but knew you needed to nourish the infant Church on earth. You lived many years with Saint John the apostle at Ephesus until our Lord took you body and soul to a place he had reserved for you at his right hand in Heaven. We honor you, Mary, Queen Assumed into Heaven.

Our Father, ten Hail Marys, Glory Be to the Father, Fatima Prayer — O my Jesus, forgive us our sins; save us from the fires of hell; lead all souls to Heaven, especially those most in need. Amen.

Our Lady of the Rosary, please obtain for me from your son the grace to not get caught up with earthly affairs and to desire Heaven above all. Pray for me that I will always set that example for my family. Please watch over my unborn child and me. Amen.

V. THE CORONATION

Dear Mother Mary, my Queen and Queen of the Universe, you are full of grace. You were crowned Queen of Heaven and Earth when you arrived in Heaven at your assumption. Your son, Jesus, has made you the mediatrix of all graces, permitting you to dispense all heavenly blessings to us. May we call upon you often. Amen.

Our Father, ten Hail Marys, Glory Be to the Father, Fatima Prayer — O my Jesus, forgive us our sins; save us from the fires of

hell; lead all souls to Heaven, especially those most in need. Amen.

Our Lady of the Rosary, please obtain for me from your son the grace of perseverance so that I may not squander my opportunities for grace throughout my lifetime so that I may finally one day take my place with the Church triumphant in Heaven. Please remind me that the prayer of the Rosary is a powerful one which I should strive to say each day. Please watch over my unborn baby and me. Amen.

* * *

A thought, a prayer, a reflection...

Queen of the most holy Rosary, pray for us.

O Mary, conceived without sin, pray for us who have recourse to thee.

VALUE OF WOMEN AS MOTHERS

Parenthood — even though it belongs to both — is realized much more fully in the woman, especially in the prenatal period. It is the woman who "pays" directly for this shared generation, which literally absorbs the energies of her body and soul. It is therefore necessary that the man be fully aware that in their shared parenthood he owes a special debt to the woman. No program of "equal rights" between women and men is valid unless it takes this fact fully into account.

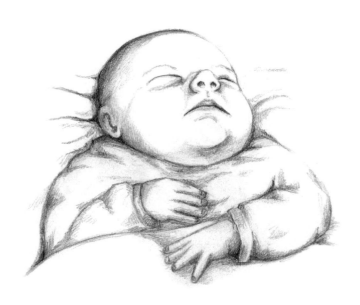

NOVENA TO
SAINT GERARD MAJELLA 3

Dear Saint Gerard, please pray for me that I may be patient with myself and others. Your example of heroic virtue in your willingness to accept everything that the Lord gave you, including the crosses, helps us all to aspire to greater holiness. Help me to remember to call upon Jesus and the Blessed Mother often throughout my pregnancy. Please watch over all expectant mothers and help my unborn baby and me. Amen.

Our Father, Hail Mary, Glory Be to the Father.
Saint Gerard, pray for us.

PRAYER FOR MY HUSBAND

Dear Jesus and Mary, when I became a mother at the conception of my child, in addition to psychological and spiritual changes, I began to undergo physical changes. My husband will not undergo the physical alterations, but in a very real way he undergoes psychological and spiritual changes because he became a father. He is no longer just a man or just a husband, but he is a father. Help me to keep in mind that he is very much a part of my pregnancy too. My husband and I are bound together in love and to our child.

Please bless him and bless me as we prepare for our little one's birth. Please help my husband see the sublimity in his role of passing on the torch of life to our child as our child blossoms within me. Amen.

PRAYER TO OUR BLESSED MOTHER

Dear Mary, my mother, thank you for caring for me, for bringing me peace and joy. Help me to love as you love and to give of myself as you do. Help me to treasure this new child within me, finding a moment here and there to relish in the miracle of life as it unfolds within me. Help me to care for this dear child with great love and devotion, now and in the future so that I may lay down the essential foundation of love and prayer in his or her life. Pray to Jesus for me, please, for all the graces I need to be a loving and patient mother. Thank you for the tender love you have for me. Hail Mary, full of grace, the Lord is with thee, blessed art thou amongst women, and blessed is the fruit of thy womb, Jesus. Holy Mary, Mother of God, pray for us sinners, now and at the hour of our death. Amen.

PRAYER FOR A FAMILY

O dear Jesus, I confidently ask you to grant my family the graces that we need to serve you well. Please, dear Lord, protect and bless all of us who are present or away, living and deceased. Help us to hold tight to each other and know that prayer will unite our hearts and souls and keep us together. Amen.

Each and every time that motherhood is repeated in human history, it is always related to the Covenant which God established with the human race through the motherhood of the Mother of God.

— POPE JOHN PAUL II, *Mulieris Dignitatem*

A GRACE-FILLED MONTH

The end of your third month has arrived. If you have been experiencing any morning sickness or nausea, you will be happy to find out that it usually begins to subside now. Your fatigue will also pretty much fade away as you regain a little more energy. You are entering your second trimester; you are a third of the way there! Perhaps you will want to get a few more things ready for your new baby as your energy level increases. But don't forget to relax too, and enjoy this most beautiful time of your life.

PRAYER FROM MY HEART

A prayer to my Lord from my heart in thanksgiving for this most beautiful gift of this new life within me:

Oh dear Lord

* * *

Reflections on My Third Month of Pregnancy

Your Fourth Month

A woman in childbirth suffers, because her time has come; but when she has given birth to the child she forgets the suffering in her joy that a human being has been born into the world.

— JOHN 16:21, NJB

The family has a special role to play throughout the life of its members, from birth to death. It is truly "the sanctuary of life: the place in which life — the gift of God — can be properly welcomed and protected against the many attacks to which it is exposed, and can develop in accordance with what constitutes authentic human growth." Consequently the role of the family in building a culture of life is decisive and irreplaceable.

— POPE JOHN PAUL II, *Evangelium Vitae*

WHAT'S HAPPENING WITH
YOUR BABY?

*D*uring the fourth month, your baby will actually grow to half the length he or she will be at birth. Your baby takes in a great deal of sustenance now, consisting of food, oxygen, and water, which are delivered through your placenta.

The placenta is the main source of hormones necessary to your body during pregnancy and helps to prepare for milk production.

Substances that enter your bloodstream will be transferred to your baby within an hour or two. This is why it is essential to only eat nourishing foods. Don't risk consuming alcohol or smoking. They are not healthy for you or for your baby. Your little one depends on you to make the appropriate decisions for proper nutrition for both of you.

At this stage of development, your unborn child has eyebrows and lashes and his or her fingers and toes are well defined. Your baby is developing reflexes and can suck a thumb and swallow.

Every child is a unique and unrepeatable gift of God, with the right to a loving and united family.

— POPE JOHN PAUL II, October 8, 1979

PRAYER TO THE HOLY FAMILY

Lord Jesus Christ, you were raised by Mary and Joseph within the Holy Family in Nazareth. Your home was humble and holy. Help us discover the holiness in simplicity and obedience to our state of life. Help us to imitate the virtues of the Holy Family as we faithfully carry out our daily duties. Please also help us to find ways to seek out solitude even in the midst of our busy lives so that we may unite our hearts with yours, dear Jesus. Please, Blessed Mother Mary and good Saint Joseph, pray for my family and protect us. Amen.

ACT OF FAITH

I firmly believe in You, my God, with all of my heart, that You are one God in three divine persons, Father, Son, and Holy Spirit. I believe that your divine son, Jesus, died for all of mankind, suffering for our sins, and I believe that he will come again to judge the living and the dead. I believe these and all the truths that our Catholic Church teaches. Thank you for the gift of faith. Please increase it in my heart. Amen.

So faith, hope, and love abide, these three; but the greatest of these is love.

— 1 CORINTHIANS 13:13, RSV (CE)

As the domestic church, the family is summoned to proclaim, celebrate and serve the Gospel of life. This is a responsibility which first concerns married couples, called to be givers of life, on the basis of an ever greater awareness of the meaning of procreation as a unique event which clearly reveals that human life is a gift received in order then to be given as a gift. In giving origin to a new life, parents recognize that the child, "as the fruit of their mutual gift of love, is, in turn, a gift for both of them, a gift which flows from them."

— POPE JOHN PAUL II, *Evangelium Vitae*

MOTHER'S DAILY PRAYER
FOR HER CHILDREN

O Mary, Immaculate Virgin, Mother of our Lord Jesus Christ, patroness of all mothers, I commend my beloved children to the Most Sacred Heart of your son, Jesus, and to your Immaculate Heart. Please assist our family and keep us always in your care. Please protect us from the snares of the devil and keep us on the road that leads to life. Help me to realize my sublime mission as a mother and help me be faithful to my duties for the good of my family and the good of the entire family of God.

Most Sacred Heart of Jesus, have mercy on us.
Immaculate Heart of Mary, pray for us.
My Guardian Angel, pray for me.
Holy Guardian Angel of our family, pray for us.
Saint Michael, pray for us.
Saint Joseph, husband of Mary, pray for us.
Saint Anne, mother of Mary, pray for us.
Saint Elizabeth, pray for us.
Saint Elizabeth Ann Seton, pray for us.
Saint Monica, pray for us.
Saint Augustine, pray for us.
Saint Gerard Majella, pray for us.
Blessed Mother Teresa of Calcutta, pray for us.
Amen.

Over all these clothes, put on love, the perfect bond.
— COLOSSIANS 3:14, NJB

PRAYER TO JESUS

Dear Jesus, thank you for the gift of my life and for the gift of the precious life within me. Help me to nurture this baby with love as it grows in my womb. In a few short months, by your grace, my baby will be in my arms to love outside my womb, to care for each day with great love and dedication. Please increase the motherly sentiments in my heart to grow more in love with my child each day so that any sacrifice I may be called to endure will be gladly borne for love of my child. Thank you, Lord, for the incredible gift of love. Amen.

Without love there is no true life in the family. Even if it passes through various difficulties, lacking things, or suffering, if love remains, the family will remain solid and united.

— POPE JOHN PAUL II, May 1, 1989

The Church stresses that every child is a human person and has the right to the integral development of his or her personality. The role of the family is irreplaceable in attaining this end, since the child cannot be understood and assisted apart from the family, which is the first educator towards physical, psychological, intellectual, moral and religious development.

— POPE PAUL VI

SPIRITUAL COMMUNION

Dear Jesus, I believe with all of my heart
that you are truly and fully present in the Blessed Sacrament.
I wish I could be near you now.
Please forgive me of all my faults.
Since I cannot receive you sacramentally at this moment,
I pray that you will come into my soul spiritually.
My heart will embrace you as you fill me with Your
    presence, Lord.
Thank you for your great love for me. Amen.

The child must be reared, educated in the family, the parents
remaining "primarily and principally responsible" for his education, a role which "is of such importance that it is almost impossible to provide an adequate substitute." That is made necessary
by the atmosphere of affection and of moral and material securi-
ty that the psychology of the child requires. It should be added
that the procreation founds this natural right, which is also "the
greatest obligation." And even the existence of wider family ties,
with brothers and sisters, with grandparents, and other close rel-
atives, is an important element which tends to be neglected
today for the child's harmonious balance.

— *Gravissimum Educationis*

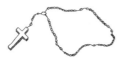

* * *

A thought, a prayer, a reflection...

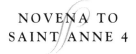

NOVENA TO
SAINT ANNE 4

Saint Anne was a woman of great hope. Her hope was rooted in an unwavering faith. Anne prayed from a humble and loving heart. On the Sabbath, she and her husband, Joachim, went to the synagogue to pray with the other faithful Jews who beseeched the heavens for the long-awaited savior. Anne gave her days over to God each morning and presented her day back to Him each night, thanking Him for her life and begging in prayer for the gift of a child one day. She never gave up hope.

PRAYER TO SAINT ANNE

Dear Saint Anne, patroness of mothers, please listen to my humble prayers to you. I ask you to continue to guide me throughout this month when my baby is growing within me. Pray to the Heavenly Father, please, to grant me the graces I most need so that I will mother my child with a pure love with all of the devotion of my heart. Guide me, please, to look for quiet moments to seek our Lord so that I will use this pregnancy wisely to be open to God's love for me and my baby in a special way. Help me to come closer to your daughter, Mary, as I pray throughout this pregnancy. Amen.

It is often regarded as the norm in our present-day society that both father and mother be employed outside the home. Such an attitude needs to be carefully reconsidered. It should be understood that the most important work a woman has to do is to provide the proper rearing and upbringing of her children. A woman who is devoted to her home and her family is, in fact, working in a very real sense and making a very real contribution to the development of the country. Let it not be thought that the process of nation building takes place only outside the home. The woman who gives her time and talents to her home and family is not depriving her family by not earning a salary. On the contrary, she is making a very significant contribution to her children in a way no money can supply.

When both parents are working away from the home, the children are often left in the care of other children. This is a twofold injustice: it is unfair to those in charge and to those who have to be tended. Even when competent persons are entrusted with the care of children, they are not adequate substitutes for the parents. The thinking should be towards providing the fathers of families with wages sufficient to support the family, so that it is not necessary for the mother to be a wage earner too.

— BISHOPS OF KENYA, Joint Pastoral Letter, 1979

DEAR MARY

Dear Mary, you are full of grace. You are the mediatrix of all grace. Please pray for me to receive the graces I am most in need of. Help me to find quiet times throughout this pregnancy to meditate and pray so that I may come closer to our Lord. Guide me, please, as I work out the details of my schedule and life ahead with my baby so that I can make arrangements to be always present to my little one, attentive to his or her needs. Please watch over me during this month of my pregnancy so that I may become who I am destined to be, by God's grace. I ask that I may live under your protective mantle. Please keep my family and all families always close to you. Amen.

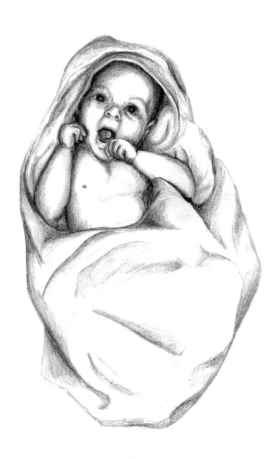

oy is not simply a matter of temperament. In the Service of God and souls, it is always hard to be joyful — all the more reason why we should try to acquire it and make it grow in our hearts.

Joy is prayer, joy is strength; joy is love; joy is a net to love by which we catch souls. God loves a cheerful giver. She gives most who gives with joy. If in the work [she is referring to the Missionaries of Charity's work, but this can be applied to all our lives] you have difficulties and you accept them with joy, with a big smile — in this, like in any other thing — they will see your good works and glorify the Father. The best way to show your gratitude is to accept everything with joy. A joyful heart is the normal result of a heart burning with love.

— BLESSED TERESA OF CALCUTTA

THE LUMINOUS MYSTERIES OF THE ROSARY

I. THE BAPTISM OF JESUS

Dear Mother Mary, when your son, Jesus, was baptized, the heavens opened wide, and he saw the Spirit of God descending like a dove and alighting on Him. A voice from Heaven cried aloud, "This is My Beloved Son with whom I am well pleased."

Our Father, ten Hail Marys, Glory Be to the Father, Fatima Prayer — O my Jesus, forgive us our sins; save us from the fires of hell; lead all souls to Heaven, especially those most in need. Amen.

Our Lady of the Rosary, please obtain for me from your son the grace to be open to the Holy Spirit in my life. Please watch over my unborn baby and me.

II. THE WEDDING AT CANA

Dear Mother Mary, you told the servants to "do whatever He tells you." Jesus told them to "fill the jars up with water." So they filled them up to the brim.

Our Father, ten Hail Marys, Glory Be to the Father, Fatima Prayer — O my Jesus, forgive us our sins; save us from the fires of hell; lead all souls to Heaven, especially those most in need. Amen.

Our Lady of the Rosary, please obtain for me from your son the grace to remember to go through you to get to Jesus. Please watch over my unborn baby and me.

III. PROCLAIMING THE KINGDOM

Dear Mother Mary, your son, Jesus, instructed the twelve disciples to go out to the lost sheep of the house of Israel and proclaim that the Kingdom of Heaven is at hand. He told them to heal the sick, raise the dead, cleanse the lepers, and drive out the demons. He told them to give without counting the cost and receiving anything in return.

Our Father, ten Hail Marys, Glory Be to the Father, Fatima Prayer — O my Jesus, forgive us our sins; save us from the fires of hell; lead all souls to Heaven, especially those most in need. Amen.

Our Lady of the Rosary, please obtain for me from your son the grace of repenting my sins often and a greater trust in God. Help me to want to give with all of my heart to help spread the word about truth and everlasting life. Please watch over my unborn baby and me.

IV. THE TRANSFIGURATION

Dear Mother Mary, your son, Jesus, was transfigured as he was praying. He became dazzling white. A voice came out of the cloud saying, "This is My Son, My chosen, listen to Him!"

Our Father, ten Hail Marys, Glory Be to the Father, Fatima Prayer — O my Jesus, forgive us our sins; save us from the fires of hell; lead all souls to Heaven, especially those most in need. Amen.

Our Lady of the Rosary, please obtain for me from your son the grace to desire holiness above all things. Please pray for my unborn baby and me.

V. THE INSTITUTION OF THE EUCHARIST

Dear Mother Mary, your son, Jesus, took bread, gave thanks, and broke it and gave it to them saying, "This is my body which is given up for you." He then took the cup after supper, saying, "This cup which is poured out for you is the new covenant in my Blood."

Our Father, ten Hail Marys, Glory Be to the Father, Fatima Prayer — O my Jesus, forgive us our sins; save us from the fires of hell; lead all souls to Heaven, especially those most in need. Amen.

Our Lady of the Rosary, please obtain for me from your son the grace to desire to come close to you in the Blessed Sacrament, where I may adore your son, Jesus, and when I cannot be there to adore him, I pray I may receive a spiritual communion. Please watch over my unborn baby and me.

Brothers, let us honor in the Birth of Christ the dawning life of man: It is a creature of God, stamped in His image and likeness (Gen. 1:16) conceived in the love, which makes of two beings, man and woman, one single life (Mark 10:8), generated, yes, not without maternal affliction, but then for the joy of the world (cf. John 16:21).

Let us honor infancy, also a creature of God, joy of the society, and called to the mysterious rebirth of Baptism, pledge of the life which shall not die.

Let us honor woman, equal with man in dignity, called to the beauty and the privileged love of consecrated virginity, or, more often, to that likewise sacrosanct love of conjugal life and to the incomparable ministry of Motherhood.

Let us honor the child, to whom the young Jesus is a brother, who, "increased in wisdom, in stature, and in favor with God and with people" (Luke 2:51, NJB).

— POPE PAUL VI, December 25, 1976

TIME TO REFLECT

Pope Paul VI reflected on the dignity of Christ and of the person in his poignant words to us. He instructs us to honor in Christ's birth "the dawning life of man." He tells us to honor man, woman, and child. He also describes the vocation of motherhood as an "incomparable ministry." Pope John Paul II has told us that love gives life to a family and that without it a family cannot survive. He said, "Even if it [the family] passes through various difficulties, lacking things, or suffering, if love remains, the family will remain solid and united." Blessed Teresa of Calcutta told us, "In the Service of God and souls, it is always hard to be joyful — all the more reason why we should try to acquire it and make it grow in our hearts." These are words we can take to our hearts and ponder as we are carrying our unborn children.

Oh Lord, show us our dignity and grant us your love as we strive to serve you in our families with joyful hearts. Amen.

NOVENA TO
SAINT GERARD MAJELLA 4

O Saint Gerard, you had to struggle to get permission to enter religious life even though you knew without a doubt that it was what God had intended for you. Circumstances caused delays and disappointments, but you remained steadfast in faith with a patient heart. Please help me during my pregnancy to be patient in all things and faithful to my state of life. Thank you for your guidance and your care in looking over me and my unborn child. Amen.

Our Father, Hail Mary, Glory Be. Saint Gerard, please pray for us.

PRAYER TO OUR BLESSED MOTHER

Oh, dear Blessed Mother Mary, the mother of my Lord and my mother too, thank you for watching over me this past month and keeping me in your care. Please continue to care for me as I continue this journey of motherhood. As my child grows inside me, help me to appreciate all the blessings that God has bestowed me with, especially for this new precious life. Hail Mary, full of grace, the Lord is with thee, blessed art thou amongst women, and blessed is the fruit of thy womb, Jesus. Holy Mary, Mother of God, pray for us sinners, now and at the hour of our death. Amen.

PRAYER FOR A FAMILY

O dear Jesus, I confidently ask you to grant my family the graces that we need to serve you well. Please, dear Lord, protect and bless all of us who are present or away, living and deceased. Help us to hold tight to each other and know that prayer will unite our hearts and souls and keep us together. Amen.

The dignity of every human being and the vocation corresponding to that dignity find their definitive measure in union with God. Mary, the woman of the Bible, is the most complete expression of this dignity and vocation. For no human being, male or female, created in the image and likeness of God, can in any way attain fulfillment apart from this image and likeness.

— POPE JOHN PAUL II, *Mulieri s Dignitatem*

A BLESSED MONTH

You and the little one hidden inside you have passed through another month of growth, both physically and spiritually. You have grown over the past weeks, and your body may now be taking on a new shape! You may have felt little flutterings and gentle movements within your womb as your little one has moved about. For some women, it is a little early to detect these movements.

It may take a little adjusting as your body changes shape. You are at an awkward stage, and you may feel some emotional ups and downs as well due to the hormonal changes in your body. It is completely natural and nothing to worry about. Have your husband put his hand on your abdomen each morning and

vening as the two of you lift your hearts and voices to Heaven
n prayer for your new baby. In addition to your daily prayers,
ind a moment here and there to lift your heart toward Heaven,
ontinuing to pray for God's grace, while enjoying this special
ime when you have been entrusted with this miraculous life
vithin you.

PRAYER FROM MY HEART

A prayer to my Lord from my heart in thanksgiving for this most
eautiful gift of new life within me:

Oh dear Lord _____

_____

_____

_____

_____

_____

_____

_____

_____

_____

_____

* * *

Reflections on My Fourth Month of Pregnancy

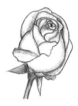

Your Fifth Month

Lo, sons are a heritage from the Lord, the
fruit of the womb a reward.
Like arrows in the hand of a warrior are
the sons of one's youth.

— PSALM 127:3–4, RSV (CE)

Motherhood always establishes a unique and unrepeatable
relationship between two people: between mother and child
and between child and mother. Even when the same woman
is the mother of many children, her personal relationship with
each one of them is of the very essence of motherhood. For
each child is generated in a unique and unrepeatable way.
And this is true both for the mother and for the child.

— POPE JOHN PAUL II, *Redemptoris Mater*

.

WHAT'S HAPPENING WITH
YOUR BABY?

*D*uring your fifth month, your baby grows in weight to a half to one pound and in length to about ten to twelve inches long. Your baby's hair also begins to grow. Your baby is now busily developing muscles and exercising them, and his or her heartbeat is louder. As your little one becomes active, you will begin to feel his or her many movements. It will feel like a fluttering to begin with. After a while and as your baby gets bigger, you will feel stronger kicks and bumping inside you. Your baby sleeps and wakes much like a newborn does. External vibrations may, at times, awaken him or her. You may notice your unborn baby moving when you are exposed to loud noises while in a movie theater, for instance, or loud music.

PRAYER TO THE HOLY FAMILY

Lord Jesus Christ, you were raised by Mary and Joseph within the Holy Family in Nazareth. Your home was humble and holy. Help us discover the holiness in simplicity and obedience to our state of life. Help us to imitate the virtues of the Holy Family as we faithfully carry out our daily duties. Please also help us to find ways to seek out solitude even in the midst of our busy lives so that we may unite our hearts with yours, dear Jesus. Please, Blessed Mother Mary and good Saint Joseph, pray for our family and protect us. Amen.

ACT OF HOPE

O dear God, I hope to obtain pardon for my sins, trusting in Your almighty and infinite mercy. I pray for Your grace and ask through Jesus Christ, my Lord and Redeemer. My hope will remain in the Lord. Amen.

MOTHER'S DAILY PRAYER
FOR HER CHILDREN

O Mary, Immaculate Virgin, Mother of our Lord Jesus Christ, patroness of all mothers, I commend my beloved children to the Most Sacred Heart of your son, Jesus, and to your Immaculate Heart. Please assist our family and keep us always in your care. Please protect us from the snares of the devil and keep us on the road that leads to life. Help me to realize my sublime mission as a mother and help me be faithful to my duties for the good of my family and the good of the entire family of God.

Most Sacred Heart of Jesus, have mercy on us.
Immaculate Heart of Mary, pray for us.
My Guardian Angel, pray for me.
Holy Guardian Angel of our family, pray for us.
Saint Michael, pray for us.
Saint Joseph, husband of Mary, pray for us.
Saint Anne, mother of Mary, pray for us.
Saint Elizabeth, pray for us.
Saint Elizabeth Ann Seton, pray for us.
Saint Monica, pray for us.

Saint Augustine, pray for us.

Saint Gerard Majella, pray for us.

Blessed Mother Teresa of Calcutta, pray for us.

Amen.

A ROYAL DESTINY

A wonderful preacher, the late Archbishop Fulton Sheen, preached that there is a royal destiny to marriage, which is a community of love as in the Trinity: to beget something outside itself. He said married couples have children because they are so in love, and since God is love, love cannot be limited. The nuptial chalice is too small for the love it contains, and therefore it must overflow. He preached that unless the couple has God in their lives, they may not desire to have children in the selfish world we live in. He tried to convey the idea that it really takes three to get married: the bride, the groom, and our Lord.

We must deepen our life of love, prayer, and sacrifice, for compassion, love, and understanding have to grow from within and from our union with Christ.

— BLESSED TERESA OF CALCUTTA

There is a tremendous strength that is growing in the world through this continual sharing together, praying together, suffering together, and working together.

— BLESSED TERESA OF CALCUTTA

*C*hristian life, a vocation which, deriving from their Baptism, has been confirmed anew and made more explicit by the Sacrament of Matrimony. For by this Sacrament they are strengthened and, one might also say, consecrated to the faithful fulfillment of their duties; to realizing to the full their vocations; and to bearing witness, as becomes them, to Christ before the world. For the Lord has entrusted to them the task of making visible to men and women the holiness, and the joy too, of the law which unites inseparably their love for one another and the cooperation they give to God's love, God who is Author of human life.

— POPE PAUL VI, *Humanae Vitae*

NOVENA TO
SAINT ANNE 5

Joachim and Anne were getting older. They still remained hopeful for a baby even at their late middle-age years. They may have begun to accept the idea that they would not receive the blessing of a child, when Anne all of a sudden found out she was pregnant. With deep joy, Anne and Joachim began to prepare their home for their baby. They were filled with peace and ever-increasing love and thankful hearts. Anne surely began to prepare little baby clothes and blankets as she prayed to the Father to fill her unborn child with grace and a holy heart to be devoted to Him in service. Then a lovely infant child was born to Anne and Joachim. Anne and Joachim beamed with happiness and thankful hearts for their gift of Mary, our Blessed Mother.

PRAYER TO SAINT ANNE

Dear Saint Anne, patroness of mothers, please listen to my humble prayers to you. I ask you to continue to guide me throughout this month when my baby is growing within me. Pray to the Heavenly Father, please, to grant me the graces I most need so that I will mother my child with a pure love and all the devotion of my heart. Help me to always hold onto hope as you have done. Guide me, please, to look for quiet moments to seek our Lord so that I will use this pregnancy wisely to be open to God's love for me and my baby in a special way. Help me to come closer to your daughter, Mary, as I pray throughout this pregnancy. Amen.

THE JOYFUL MYSTERIES
OF THE ROSARY
(See above pages 33–37)

I. The Annunciation

II. The Visitation

III. The Nativity

IV. Presentation of the Child Jesus in the Temple

V. Finding the Child Jesus in the Temple

A BRIGHTLY BURNING TORCH

We have no wish at all to pass over in silence the difficulties, at times very great, which beset the lives of Christian married couples. For them, as indeed for every one of us, "the gate is narrow and the way is hard that leads to life" (cf. Matt. 7:14). Nevertheless it is precisely the hope of that life which, like a brightly burning torch, lights up their journey, as, strong in spirit, they strive to live "sober, upright, and godly lives in this world" (cf. Tim. 2:12) knowing for sure that "the form of this world is passing away" (cf. 1 Cor.7:31).

— POPE PAUL VI, *Humanae Vitae*

Woman both as a person and as a mother derives all of her dignity from God and His wise dispositions. As a result, natural law makes it an inalienable and inviolable dignity which women are obliged to preserve, protect, and increase.

— POPE PIUS XII, October 14, 1956

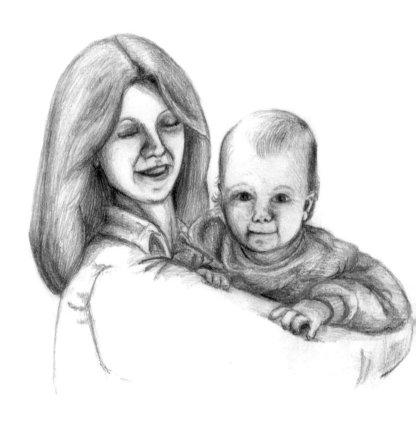

NOVENA TO
SAINT GERARD MAJELLA 5

Dear Saint Gerard, you were very devoted to the Eucharist. Please pray for me to have the grace to understand the profound and living faith in the great mystery of the Blessed Sacrament. Please remind me that I am in the company of God Himself, I am with Jesus, my Lord, who is present totally — body, blood, soul, and divinity. Help me to appreciate this great gift of the Eucharist, and inspire me to long to be near Jesus whenever I can, bringing my children to him, too. When I am not able to receive him in Holy Communion, please remind me to ask him to come into my heart spiritually to nourish my soul and fill me with his presence so I may radiate him to my family and others. Amen.

Our Father, Hail Mary, Glory Be. Saint Gerard, please pray for us.

SPIRITUAL COMMUNION

Dear Jesus, I believe with all of my heart
that you are truly and fully present in the Blessed Sacrament.
I wish I could be near you now.
Please forgive me of all my faults.
Since I cannot receive you sacramentally at this moment,
I pray that you will come into my soul spiritually. My heart will
embrace you as you fill me with Your presence, Lord.
Thank you for your great love for me. Amen.

* * *

A thought, a prayer, a reflection...

PRAYER TO OUR BLESSED MOTHER

Dear Blessed Mother Mary, thank you for guiding me through this month of pregnancy. Please help me to be more prayerful. Help me to look to your son, Jesus, often. Please pray for me to receive the graces that I am in most need of.

Please help me so that I will want to imitate you in your holiness, purity, humility, love, and grace. I pray I can be a good mother; help me to please attain that goal. Thank you for the beautiful love you have for me and for my unborn baby. Hail Mary, full of grace, the Lord is with thee, blessed art thou amongst women, and blessed is the fruit of thy womb, Jesus. Holy Mary, Mother of God, pray for us sinners, now and at the hour of our death. Amen.

PRAYER FOR A FAMILY

O dear Jesus, I confidently ask you to grant my family the graces that we need to serve you well. Please, dear Lord, protect and bless all of us who are present or away, living and deceased. Help us to hold tight to each other and know that prayer will unite our hearts and souls and keep us together. Amen.

A GRACE-FILED MONTH

The end of your fifth month — wow! You are more than halfway there! Hopefully you have been able to find some quiet time during this month to rest and meditate as you have felt your precious one moving inside you. Be sure to take the time to jot down your thoughts, prayers, and reflections as you journey through this pregnancy. You will have a memorable keepsake of your baby's beginnings. Pray often to our Lord and his Blessed Mother as they guide you through your pregnancy. Spend time with your husband when possible; when your child is born, you will be very busy for a while, adjusting to a new schedule and trying to keep up with the demands of motherhood, as well as attempting to get some rest whenever you can. Pray with your husband each morning and each evening for your unborn child.

PRAYER FROM MY HEART

A prayer to my Lord from my heart in thanksgiving for this most beautiful gift of new life within me:

Oh dear Lord _____

_____

_____

_____

_____

* * *

Reflections on My Fifth Month of Pregnancy

Your Sixth Month

By the mouths of children, babes in arms, you have made sure of praise?

— MATTHEW 21:16b, NJB

Our total surrender will come today by surrendering even our sins so that we will be poor. "Unless you become a child you cannot come to me." You are too big, too heavy, you cannot be lifted up. We need humility to acknowledge our sin. The knowledge of our sin helps us to rise. I will get up and go to my Father.

— BLESSED TERESA OF CALCUTTA

WHAT'S HAPPENING WITH
YOUR BABY?

This sixth month, your baby will grow about two more inches to become about fourteen inches long and will grow to weigh between one and a half and two pounds. He or she will also begin to accumulate a little fat under the skin. During this month, the buds for permanent teeth will come in, high in the gums behind the milk teeth. Your baby can now open his or her closed eyelids and may look up, down, and sideways. With continued muscle development your baby will now have a strong grip. If born prematurely, your baby could maintain regular breathing for about twenty-four hours.

An incubator with intensive care would support a chance of survival at this point. Your baby's skin is reddish in color, wrinkled, and covered with a heavy, protective, creamy coating called vernix caeosa.

By the end of the sixth month your baby will have completed two-thirds of his or her stay in your womb.

PRAYER TO THE HOLY FAMILY

Lord Jesus Christ, you were raised by Mary and Joseph within the Holy Family in Nazareth. Your home was humble and holy. Help us discover the holiness in simplicity and obedience to our state of life. Help us to imitate the virtues of the Holy Family as we faithfully carry out our daily duties. Please also help us to find ways to seek out solitude even in the midst of our busy lives so that we may unite our hearts with yours, dear Jesus. Please, Blessed Mother Mary and good Saint Joseph, pray for us and protect us. Amen.

ACT OF FAITH

I firmly believe in You, my God, with all of my heart, that You are one God in three divine persons, Father, Son, and Holy Spirit. I believe that your divine son, Jesus, died for all of mankind, suffering for our sins, and I believe that he will come again to judge the living and the dead. I believe these and all the truths that our Catholic Church teaches. Thank you for the gift of faith. Please increase it in my heart. Amen.

MOTHER'S DAILY PRAYER
FOR HER CHILDREN

O Mary, Immaculate Virgin, Mother of our Lord Jesus Christ, patroness of all mothers, I commend my beloved children to the Most Sacred Heart of your son, Jesus, and to your Immaculate Heart. Please assist our family and keep us always in your care. Please protect us from the snares of the devil and keep us on the road that leads to life. Help me to realize my sublime mission as a mother and help me be faithful to my duties for the good of my family and the good of the entire family of God.

Most Sacred Heart of Jesus, have mercy on us.
Immaculate Heart of Mary, pray for us.
My Guardian Angel, pray for me.

Holy Guardian Angel of our family, pray for us.
Saint Michael, pray for us.
Saint Joseph, husband of Mary, pray for us.
Saint Anne, mother of Mary, pray for us.
Saint Elizabeth, pray for us.
Saint Elizabeth Ann Seton, pray for us.
Saint Monica, pray for us.
Saint Augustine, pray for us.
Saint Gerard Majella, pray for us.
Blessed Mother Teresa of Calcutta, pray for us.
Amen.

We learn from Saint Augustine, who was considered one of the greatest experts of the human heart, "Our freedom consists in our subjection to the truth." Our Church teaches us to forever seek the truth, to venerate it and obey it. We shall not go wrong when we sincerely search with a pure heart and fully obey God's truth. According to Blessed Teresa of Calcutta, living the Truth sets us free.

* * *

A thought, a prayer, a reflection...

LEARNING TO PRAY WITH HUMILITY

Where can I learn to pray? Jesus taught us: "Pray like this: Our Father, Thy will be done. Forgive us as we forgive." It is so simple yet so beautiful. If we pray the "Our Father" and live it, we will be holy. Everything is there: God, myself, my neighbor. If I forgive, then I can be holy and can pray all this comes from a humble heart, and if we have this we will know how to love God, to love self, and to love your neighbor.

This is not complicated, and yet we complicate our lives so much, by so many additions. Just one thing counts: to be humble, to pray. The more you pray, the better you will pray. How do you pray? You should go to God like a little child. A child has no difficulty expressing his little mind in simple words, which say so much. Jesus said to Nicodemus: "Become as a little child." If we pray the gospel, we will allow Christ to grow in us.

One thing is necessary for us — confession. Confession is nothing but humility in action. We used to call it penance, but really it is a sacrament of love, a sacrament of forgiveness. That is why confession should not be a place in which to talk for long hours about our difficulties. It is a place where I allow Jesus to take away from me everything that divides, that destroys. Where there is a gap between Christ, and me when my love is divided, anything can come to fill the gap. We should be very simple and childlike in confession. "Here I am as a child going to her Father." If a child is not yet spoiled and has not learned to tell lies, he will tell everything. This is what I mean by being childlike. Confession is a beautiful act of great love. Only in confession can we go as sinners with sin and come out as sinners without sin.

— BLESSED TERESA OF CALCUTTA

NOVENA TO
SAINT ANNE 6

Along with the birth of our Blessed Mother Mary came sweetness beyond description for her parents, Anne and Joachim. Their humble household was filled with love and peace. Anne and Joachim felt gloriously fulfilled with the precious gift that God had bestowed upon them.

Their days were filled with ordinary occurrences and routines marked with extraordinary grace. Mary learned from parents, who were eager to teach their child the truth about life, God's laws, and His great love for mankind. Mary learned from her parents about the savior that her people had been awaiting. She became well-informed about the dignity in a mother's work in the home, caring for the household, by watching her mother, Anne.

Anne and Joachim were thankful that their trust and hope in God's providence for a child was not in vain.

PRAYER TO SAINT ANNE

Dear Saint Anne, patroness of mothers, please listen to my humble prayers to you. I ask you to continue to guide me throughout this month when my baby is growing within me. Pray to the Heavenly Father, please, to grant me the graces I most need so that I will mother my child with a pure love and all the devotion of my heart. Help me to always hold onto hope as you have done. Guide me, please, to look for quiet moments to seek our Lord so that I will use this pregnancy wisely to be open to God's love for me and my baby in a special way. Help me to come closer to your daughter, Mary, as I pray throughout this pregnancy. Amen.

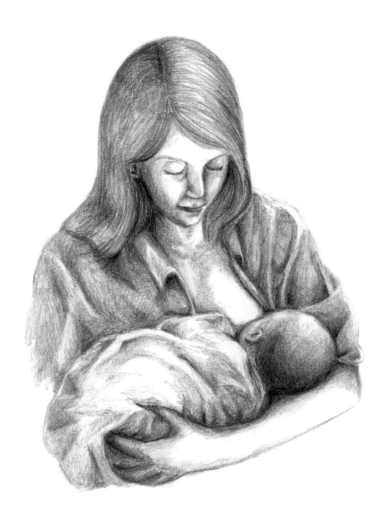

From the moment a child is conceived, as geneticists tell us, he is endowed with his own characteristics of a life which is no less autonomous for the fact that he be tributary to a privileged environment of development.

— SECRETARY OF STATE J. CARDINAL VILLOT,
IN THE NAME OF THE HOLY FATHER, OCTOBER 3, 1970

THE SORROWFUL MYSTERIES
OF THE ROSARY
(See above pages 50–54)

I. The Agony in the Garden
II. The Scourging at the Pillar
III. The Crowning with Thorns
IV. The Carrying of the Cross
V. The Crucifixion

WOMEN AS A SOURCE OF STRENGTH

A woman is strong because of her awareness of this entrusting, strong because of the fact that God "entrusts the human being to her" always and in every way, even in the situations of social discrimination in which she may find herself. This awareness and this fundamental vocation speak to women of the dignity which they receive from God himself, and this makes them "strong" and strengthens their vocation.

Thus the "perfect woman" (cf. Prov 31:10) becomes an irreplaceable support and source of spiritual strength for other people, who perceive the great energies of her spirit. These "perfect women" are owed much by their families, and sometimes by whole nations.

— JOHN PAUL II, *Mulieris Dignitatem*

PRAYER TO JESUS

Dear Jesus, I am in absolute awe when I look down and see my protruding abdomen. I have been feeling life within me, which is truly a miracle to behold. I thank you, Lord, from the deepest part of my heart for this precious gift of life that you have blessed me with. Thank you for the amazing call you have given me to raise this child. Help me to teach my child to be confident with his or her unique personal dignity. I pray that I can always treasure this new life and nurture it beyond measure throughout all his or her days until we come face to face with you in Heaven one day. Amen.

A RECIPROCAL DONATION OF SELF

There has forever been a bone of contention between man and woman or at least a general misunderstanding throughout the ages about whether or not a wife should be subject to her husband. Even among the well-intentioned there are disagreements in this regard. Men may feel that they can and should "lord" over their wives and be served by them, whereas women may feel that they should be "beneath" their husbands or may feel resentful when thought of as only a servant by their husbands.

When we read the letter to the Ephesians 5:21–23, we see that the author is addressing husbands and wives and instructs them to be subject to one another out of reverence for Christ. The words in this letter to the Ephesians, when taken out of context can wreak all kinds of havoc.

Pope John Paul II made sure he addressed all of this in "The Theology of Marriage and Celibacy." He said, "The opening expression of our passage of Ephesians 5:21–23, which we have approached by an analysis of the remote and immediate context, has quite a special eloquence. The author speaks of the mutual subjection of the spouses, husband and wife, and in this way he explains the words which he will unite afterwards on the subjection of the spouses, husband and wife. In fact we read; 'Wives be subject to your husbands, as to the Lord' (5:22, RSV [CE]). In saying this, the author does not intend to say that the husband is the 'lord' of the wife and that the interpersonal pact proper to marriage is a pact of domination of the husband over the wife. Instead, he expresses a different concept: that is, that the wife can and should find in her relationship with Christ, who is the one Lord of both the spouses — the motivation of that relationship with her husband which flows from the very essence of marriage and of the family. Such a relationship, however, is not one of one-sided domination. Marriage, according to the letter to the Ephesians, excludes the element of the pact, which was a burden and, at times, does not cease to be a burden on this institution. The husband and the wife are in fact 'subject to one another' and are mutually subordinated to one another. The source of this mutual subjection is to be found in Christian pietas, and its expression is love.

"Love excludes every kind of subjection whereby the wife might become a servant or a slave of the husband, an object of unilateral domination. Love makes the husband simultaneously subject to the wife, and thereby subject to the Lord Himself, ju. as the wife to the husband. The community or unity, which the should establish through marriage, is constituted by a reciprocal donation of self, which is also a mutual subjection. Christ is the source and at the same time the model of that subjection, which being reciprocal 'out of reverence for Christ,' confers on the conjugal union a profound and mature character" (Pope John Paul II, General Audience of August 11, 1982).

NOVENA TO
SAINT GERARD MAJELLA 6

Dear Saint Gerard, you are known for living in the spirit of the "Our Father" and for forgiving others always, even in the face of false accusations. Please pray that I will also be an instrument of peace for our Lord. Please pray that I will receive all of the graces I am most in need of. Guide me through my pregnancy. Amen.

Our Father, Hail Mary, Glory Be.
Saint Gerard, please pray for us.

SPIRITUAL COMMUNION

Dear Jesus, I believe with all of my heart
that you are truly and fully present in the Blessed Sacrament.
I wish I could be near you now.
Please forgive me all of my faults.
Since I cannot receive you sacramentally at this moment,
I pray that you will come into my soul spiritually. My heart will embrace you as you fill me with your presence, Lord.
Thank you for Your great love for me. Amen.

PRAYER TO OUR BLESSED MOTHER

Dear Blessed Mother Mary; you have taken me through another month of pregnancy, a most privileged time during my life. Please help me to grow closer to you and your son, Jesus. Please pray for me and inspire me to grow in my faith. Help me to recognize that there are times throughout my busy schedule when I can fit in prayer even in bits and pieces and times for reading spiritual writings, including the Bible, to help nourish my faith. Help me to find the proper balance between my family activities, care of my home and family, and my prayer life. Help me to be content with the beautiful vocation of motherhood that God has gifted me with. Hail Mary, full of grace, the Lord is with thee, blessed art thou amongst women, and blessed is the fruit of thy womb, Jesus.

Holy Mary, Mother of God, pray for us sinners, now and at the hour of our death. Amen.

PRAYER FOR A FAMILY

O dear Jesus, I confidently ask you to grant my family the graces that we need to serve you well. Please, dear Lord, protect and bless all of us who are present or away, living and deceased. Help us to hold tight to each other and know that prayer will unite our hearts and souls and keep us together. Amen.

A BLESSED MONTH

Your sixth month of pregnancy has come to a close. Take some time to reflect on the past month. Your size and shape have been ever-changing. You undoubtedly have been feeling much more movement from your little one. Be sure to enjoy the gentle flutters and bumps as your baby flips and turns in your womb, your child's God-given home. These delightful moments, realizing the life within you, will remain with you as fond memories in times ahead. Encourage your husband to partake in this joy, placing his hand on your abdomen to experience the movements. Speak to your baby. He or she will recognize your voice when you meet each other face to face. Pray for your little one each day, even before he or she has seen the light of day.

PRAYER FROM MY HEART

A prayer to my Lord from my heart in thanksgiving for this most beautiful gift of this new life within me:

Oh dear Lord _____

_____

_____

_____

_____

* * *

Reflections on My Sixth Month of Pregnancy

Your Seventh Month

You created my inmost self,
knit me together in my mother's womb.
For so many marvels I thank you;
a wonder am I, and all your works are wonders. You knew
me through and through.

— PSALM 139:13–14, NJB

The basic need of any child is a family where both parents
cooperate harmoniously in its upbringing. Both parents have
the right and the duty to devote themselves to the rearing and
the education of the children they are responsible for having
brought into the world. Where either parent neglects his (her)
duty, a serious wrong is done to the other parent and the
child.

— BISHOPS OF KENYA, JOINT PASTORAL LETTER 1979

We know this is not always possible, such as in the case of a single-parent household, but when two parents are present, a mother and father should encourage one another to give of themselves wholeheartedly, working together to raise their children in the best way possible. It will be work that is priceless.

WHAT'S HAPPENING WITH YOUR BABY?

Your baby will most likely put on more than a pound during his or her seventh month in your womb. Fat deposits build up and hair may grow long. Your baby may suck his or her thumb, hiccup, and respond to stimuli, including pain, light, and sound. During this month, your baby will continue to exercise. The volume of amniotic fluid will begin to diminish as your baby takes up more space in your womb. If your baby is born in the last part of this month, he or she will have a good chance for survival with skilled intensive care.

PRAYER TO THE HOLY FAMILY

Lord Jesus Christ, you were raised by Mary and Joseph within the Holy Family in Nazareth. Your home was humble and holy. Help us discover the holiness in simplicity and obedience to our state of life. Help us to imitate the virtues of the Holy Family. Please also help us to find ways to seek out solitude even in the midst of our busy lives so that we may unite our hearts with yours, dear Jesus. Please, Blessed Mother Mary and good Saint Joseph, pray for my family and protect us. Amen.

ACT OF FAITH

I firmly believe in You, my God, with all of my heart, that You are one God in three divine persons, Father, Son, and Holy Spirit. I believe that your divine son, Jesus, died for all of mankind, suffering for our sins, and I believe that he will come again to judge the living and the dead. I believe these and all the truths that our Catholic Church teaches. Thank you for the gift of faith. Please increase it in my heart. Amen.

MOTHER'S DAILY PRAYER
FOR HER CHILDREN

O Mary, Immaculate Virgin, Mother of our Lord Jesus Christ, patroness of all mothers, I commend my beloved children to the Most Sacred Heart of your son, Jesus, and to your Immaculate Heart. Please assist our family and keep us always in your care. Please protect us from the snares of the devil and keep us on the road that leads to life. Help me to realize my sublime mission as a mother and help me be faithful to my duties for the good of my family and the good of the entire family of God.

Most Sacred Heart of Jesus, have mercy on us.
Immaculate Heart of Mary, pray for us.
My Guardian Angel, pray for me.
Holy Guardian Angel of our family, pray for us.
Saint Michael, pray for us.

Saint Joseph, husband of Mary, pray for us.
Saint Anne, mother of Mary, pray for us.
Saint Elizabeth, pray for us.
Saint Elizabeth Ann Seton, pray for us.
Saint Monica, pray for us.
Saint Augustine, pray for us.
Saint Gerard Majella, pray for us.
Blessed Mother Teresa of Calcutta, pray for us. Amen.

PRAY WITH YOUR HEART

"Pray constantly" (1 Thess. 5:17, NJB). Take the time to pray whenever you can. Praying is not just words, but sentiments from the heart — a sincere desire to come closer to our Lord by giving of oneself from the heart. Go about your days raising your heart to the Lord and his Mother Mary, asking them for help and grace in your vocation as a mother and thanking them for their great love for us. When you pause occasionally, turning your focus from your ordinary daily activities and raising your heart in prayer, our Lord will hear you and will speak to your heart. You have to train yourself to listen to him.

Blessed Teresa of Calcutta said, "A soul of prayer can make progress without recourse to words, by learning to listen, to be present to Christ, and to look towards Him." This progress of growing in holiness that Blessed Teresa spoke of is a benefit not only to you, but to your family and your neighbor as well.

You can draw encouragement from the words of Saint John Chrysostom, who said, "It is possible to offer fervent prayer even while walking in public or strolling alone, or seated in your shop, while buying or selling, or even while cooking" ("Ecloga de oratione" 2: PG 63, 585). Saint Alphonsus Liguori said, "Those who pray are certainly saved; those who do not pray are certainly damned" (Del gran mezzo della preghiera).

"He [she] prays 'without ceasing' who unites prayer to works and good works to prayer. Only in this way can we consider as realizable the principal of praying without ceasing" (Origen, De orat. 12: PG 11, 452C).

Draw away from the hubbub clamoring for your attention as best as you can, retreating to your heart as often as you are able. And when it is impossible to draw away because of the need to be immersed in the job at hand, offer your heart to the Lord throughout all of it. By offering your days to the Lord when you open your eyes to a new day, each day, you will remain in communication with our Lord. Let us pray that our very lives will become an unceasing prayer.

PRAYER OF CONSECRATION

Dear Mother Mary, before my baby even sees the light of day, I consecrate him or her to you. I am truly blessed to be carrying this baby within my womb. This is my child, but more accurately he or she belongs to the Lord. I pray for your grace, Mother Mary, to consecrate my baby into the Lord's service. Help me guide my child in the truth with a firm belief in him who is the Truth, in purity because my child's body is a temple of God, and in sacrifice because Jesus Christ died for his or her sins. You presented your child, Jesus, in the Temple for the world's redemption. I consecrate my child to you, dear Mother Mary, to fulfill my duty as a mother in the care of this little soul who is entrusted to my care. Amen.

While the dignity of woman witnesses to the love which she receives in order to love in return, the biblical "exemplar" of the Woman also seems to reveal *the true order of love which constitutes woman's own vocation*. Vocation is meant here in its fundamental, and one may say universal significance, a significance which is then actualized and expressed in woman's many different "vocations" in the Church and the world.

— JOHN PAUL II, *Mulieri s Dignitatem*

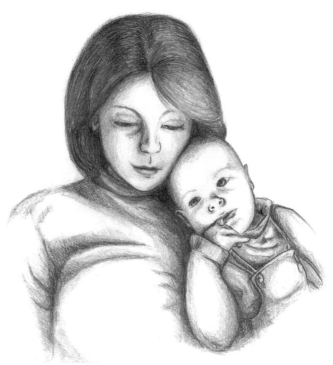

NOVENA TO
SAINT ANNE 7

It is not known whether Anne was alive when baby Jesus was born to Mary. From the silence of the Scriptures, we are led to believe that she already may have gone home to God. Undoubtedly, the spirit of Anne's devotedness, loving kindnesses, and virtuous patience lived on in Mary. Blessed Mother Mary learned the art of mothering from her mother, Anne. Mary in turn passed down to her son, Jesus, the teachings she had learned from her mother's knee, her Jewish faith, and the words of the prophets. Jesus grew in wisdom and grace in the humble household of Mary and Joseph.

PRAYER TO SAINT ANNE

Dear Saint Anne, patroness of mothers, please listen to my humble prayers to you. I ask you to continue to guide me throughout this month when my baby is growing within me. Pray to the Heavenly Father, please, to grant me the graces I most need so that I will mother my child with a pure love and all the devotion of my heart. Help me to always hold onto hope as you have done. Guide me, please, to look for quiet moments to seek our Lord so that I will use this pregnancy wisely to be open to God's love for me and my baby in a special way. Help me to come closer to your daughter, Mary, as I pray throughout this pregnancy. Amen.

woman's dignity is closely connected with the love which she receives by the very reason of her femininity; it is likewise connected with the love which she gives in return. The truth about the person and about love is thus confirmed with regard to the truth about the person, we must turn again to the Second Vatican Council: "Man, who is the only creature on earth that God willed for its own sake, cannot fully find himself except through a sincere gift of self." This applies to every human being, as a person created in God's image, whether man or woman. This ontological affirmation also indicated the ethical dimension of a person's vocation. Woman can only find herself by giving love to others.

— POPE JOHN PAUL II, *Mulieri s Dignitatem*

THE GLORIOUS MYSTERIES
OF THE ROSARY
(See above pages 67–71)

I. The Resurrection
II. The Ascension
III. The Descent of the Holy Spirit
IV. The Assumption
V. The Coronation

LITTLE THINGS

Being a mother means that your days may be filled with many little things that you do — small acts of love and service to your family members and others. Some people may look upon a mother's role or a mother's actions within her family or household as mundane or unimportant. Saint Thérèse of Lisieux was known for her "little way of love." She believed in doing everything simply and lovingly to please our Lord. She possessed an unshakeable, childlike faith.

We can also learn a lot from Saint Augustine, who said, "Little things are indeed little, but to be faithful in little things is a great thing." Blessed Teresa of Calcutta also knew the great value in little things. She said, "Be faithful in little things, for in them our strength lies. To the good God nothing is little because He is great and we are small."

So, while you go about your days as a mother, doing your little things, don't feel that your role is little or insignificant, rather know in your heart that God sees all of the ordinary little things you do with extraordinary love and blesses you in a big way for it.

NOVENA TO
SAINT GERARD MAJELLA 7

Dear Saint Gerard Majella, I trust in your powerful intercession before the Blessed Trinity. I present my request to you now as I am carrying my baby. Please also pray for the graces I need to be the mother I should be. Please pray that God will instill within my heart the same love that you had for God's holy will. Please guide me and watch over my baby and me. Amen.

SPIRITUAL COMMUNION

Dear Jesus, I believe with all of my heart
That you are truly and fully present in the Blessed Sacrament.
I wish I could be near you now.
Please forgive me all of my faults.
Since I cannot receive you sacramentally at this moment,
I pray that you will come into my soul spiritually. My heart
    will embrace you as you fill me with your presence, Lord.
Thank you for your great love for me. Amen.

* * *

A thought, a prayer, a reflection...

*T*he well-being of the individual person and of human and Christian society is intimately linked with the healthy condition of the communion set up by marriage and the family. We are all aware of certain contemporary trends which seem to threaten the stability, if not the very existence, of the family: a shift of emphasis toward the comfort of the individual over the well-being of the family as society's basic social unit, increasing divorce rates, attitudes of sexual permissiveness and the suggestion that other types of relationships can replace marriage and the family.

We simply cannot accept the contemporary pursuit of exaggerated convenience and comfort, for as Christians we must heed the vigorous exhortation of Saint Paul: "Do not be conformed to this world... " (Romans 12:2, RSV [CE]). We must realize that in our struggles to overcome the negative influences of modern society we are identified with Christ the Lord, who by His suffering and death has redeemed the world.

— POPE JOHN PAUL II, September 24, 1983

PRAYER TO OUR BLESSED MOTHER

Oh, dear Blessed Mother, thank you once again for guiding me safely through another month of pregnancy. My thoughts sometimes turn to your pregnancy with Jesus, and I try to fathom how you must have felt carrying your son in your womb. I'm sure you experienced the same joy as I experience now when my baby stirs, knowing there is a precious life within me! Please pray for me now and throughout the remainder of my pregnancy. Pray that my husband and I will remain close and understanding of each other. Keep us prayerful and loving so we may be good parents as we raise our child in love and truth. Help us, dear Mary, to prepare for our baby's arrival. Hail Mary, full of grace, the Lord is with thee, blessed are thou amongst women, and blessed is the fruit of thy womb, Jesus. Holy Mary, Mother of God, pray for us sinners, now and at the hour of our death. Amen

PRAYER FOR A FAMILY

O dear Jesus, I confidently ask you to grant my family the graces that we need to serve you well. Please, dear Lord, protect and bless all of us who are present or away, living and deceased. Help us to hold tight to each other and know that prayer will unite our hearts and souls and keep us together. Amen.

A GRACE-FILLED MONTH

With two months to go, you must be getting pretty excited and also very busy as you prepare for your little one's arrival. You may be getting your little one's crib or cradle and clothes ready. It's a wonderful time of joyful expectation! Mothers are privileged to partake in God's creation of a new life. You may also be somewhat uncomfortable as you grow bigger and bigger! You cannot get around as easily as before. Slow down a little so you can enjoy this time. Don't fret about the inconveniences due to your shape and your baby growing inside you. Rest when you can, and look forward to meeting that bundle of love and joy that awaits you! Thank God for this very precious gift.

PRAYER FROM MY HEART

A prayer to my Lord from my heart in Thanksgiving for this most beautiful gift of new life within me.

Oh dear Lord _____

_____

_____

_____

_____

_____

* * *

Reflections on My Seventh Month of Pregnancy

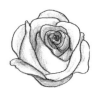

Your Eighth Month

For thou, O Lord, art my hope,
my trust, O Lord, from my youth.
Upon thee I have leaned from my birth;
thou art he who took me from my mother's womb. My praise
is continually of thee.
I have been as a portent to many;
but thou art my strong refuge.
My mouth is filled with thy praise,
and with thy glory all the day.

— PSALM 71:5–8, RSV (CE)

I wish to express the joy that we all find in children, the springtime of life, the anticipation of the future history of each of our present earthly homelands. No country on earth, no political system can think of its own future other than through the image of these new generations that will receive from their parents the manifold heritage of values, duties and aspirations of the nation of which they belong and of the whole human family.

Concern for the child, even before birth, from the first moment of conception and then throughout the years of infancy and youth, is the primary and fundamental test of the relationship of one human being to another.

— POPE JOHN PAUL II, October 2, 1979, at the United Nations

WHAT'S HAPPENING WITH YOUR BABY?

During the eighth month, your baby will gain at least two pounds. It will be mostly a protective padding of fat that will help keep your baby warm after birth. By the end of this month, he or she will fit snugly in your womb and he will no longer be able to flip and do somersaults, only turning from side to side. Usually during this time a baby settles in a head-down position, because the head is heaviest and fits into the bottom contour of the uterus. Your baby is now about eighteen inches long and will weigh at least five pounds. His or her lungs are now mature.

PRAYER TO THE HOLY FAMILY

Lord Jesus Christ, you were raised by Mary and Joseph within the Holy Family in Nazareth. Your home was humble and holy. Help us discover the holiness in simplicity and obedience to our state of life. Help us to imitate the virtues of the Holy Family. Please also help us to find ways to seek out solitude even in the midst of our busy lives so that we may unite our hearts with yours, dear Jesus. Please, Blessed Mother Mary and good Saint Joseph, pray for us and protect us. Amen.

ACT OF HOPE

O dear God, I hope to obtain pardon for my sins, trusting in your almighty and infinite mercy. I pray for your grace and ask for grace through Jesus Christ, my Lord and Redeemer. My hope will remain in the Lord. Amen.

MOTHER'S DAILY PRAYER
FOR HER CHILDREN

O Mary, Immaculate Virgin, Mother of our Lord Jesus Christ, patroness of all mothers, I commend my beloved children to the Most Sacred Heart of your son, Jesus, and to your Immaculate Heart. Please assist our family and keep us always in your care. Please protect us from the snares of the devil and keep us on the road that leads to life. Help me to realize my sublime mission as a mother and help me be faithful to my duties for the good of my family and the good of the entire family of God.

Most Sacred Heart of Jesus, have mercy on us.
Immaculate Heart of Mary, pray for us.

My Guardian Angel, pray for me.

Holy Guardian Angel of our family, pray for us.

Saint Michael, pray for us.

Saint Joseph, husband of Mary, pray for us.

Saint Anne, mother of Mary, pray for us.

Saint Elizabeth, pray for us.

Saint Elizabeth Ann Seton, pray for us.

Saint Monica, pray for us.

Saint Augustine, pray for us.

Saint Gerard Majella, pray for us.

Blessed Mother Teresa of Calcutta, pray for us. Amen.

PRAYER TO CORRECT MY CHILDREN PROPERLY

Dear Lord, Jesus, please grant me the graces I need to always correct my children with love. Saint Paul expressed, "You who are fathers, do not rouse your children to resentment; the training, the disciplines in which you bring them up must come from the Lord." Help me to remember that discipline and authority do not mean exasperating or provoking my children. I know that raising children takes a patient, loving, and diligent parent. Please help me to continually be sensitive to the unique personalities of my children. I pray that I will never correct my children in anger and that I will never abuse my parental power, but will instead correct in the spirit of the Lord. I know, too, that if I do not shepherd my children according to your ways, Lord, the devil will take over and lead my children down the path to destruction. Please grant me the gift of discernment and give me your peace in my vocation of love as I guide my children to you. Amen.

NOVENA TO
SAINT ANNE 8

In years past, the names of Mary and Anne were considered to be the most honorable for a girl or a woman. Motherly virtues come to mind, which are intimately associated with these two beautiful names.

Today the names of Mary and Anne remain symbols of strength and power. When we call upon Anne, we know that Jesus will undoubtedly listen to his devoted grandmother's prayers, interceding on our behalf.

PRAYER TO SAINT ANNE

Dear Saint Anne, patroness of mothers, please listen to my humble prayers to you. I ask you to continue to guide me throughout this month when my baby is growing within me. Pray to the Heavenly Father, please, to grant me the graces I most need so that I will mother my child with a pure love and all the devotion of my heart. Guide me, please, to look for quiet moments to seek our Lord so that I will use this pregnancy wisely to be open to God's love for me and my baby in a special way. Help me to come closer to your daughter, Mary, as I pray throughout this pregnancy. Amen.

PRAYER TO OUR DEAR LORD

Thank you, dear Lord God, for creating our family and giving us our unique identity. Please grant us the graces, dear Jesus and

Mary, to accept our dynamic role and to realize our calling to a lofty responsibility, never to ignore what we are being called to do to further the Kingdom. Help us to be always open to one another with an abundance of love, understanding, forbearance, and pardon. Please keep us united in your love as we learn to become who we are. Amen.

OUR UNIQUE IDENTITY

Above all it is important to underline the equal dignity and responsibility of women and men. This equality is realized in a unique manner in that reciprocal self-giving by each one to the other and by both to the children, which is proper to marriage and family. What human reason intuitively perceives and acknowledges is fully revealed by the word of God: the history of salvation, in fact, is a continuous and luminous testimony to the dignity of women.

In creating the human race "male and female," God gives man and woman an equal personal dignity, endowing them with the inalienable rights and responsibilities proper to the human person. God then manifests the dignity of women in the highest form possible, by assuming human flesh from the Virgin Mary, whom the Church honors as the Mother of God, calling her the new Eve and presenting her as the model of redeemed woman. The sensitive respect of Jesus towards the women that he called to his following and friendship, his appearing on Easter morning to a woman before the other disciples, the mission entrusted to women to carry the Good News of the Resurrection to the Apostles — these are all the signs that confirm the special esteem of the Lord Jesus for women. The Apostle Paul will say: "In Christ Jesus you are all children of God through faith. There is neither Jew nor Greek, there is neither slave nor free, there is neither male nor female for you are all one in Christ Jesus."

— POPE JOHN PAUL II, *Familiaris Consortio*

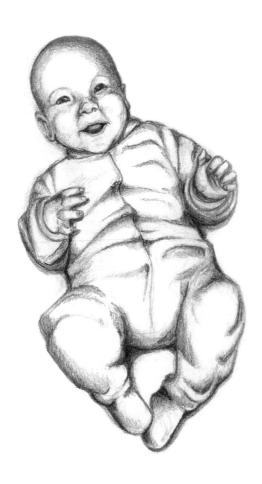

THE SORROWFUL MYSTERIES OF THE ROSARY

(See above pages 50–54)

I. The Agony in the Garden
II. The Scourging at the Pillar
III. The Crowning with Thorns
IV. The Carrying of the Cross
V. The Crucifixion

While it must be recognized that women have the same right as men to perform various public functions, society must be structured in such a way that wives and mothers *are not in practice compelled* to work outside the home, and that their families can live and prosper in a dignified way even when they themselves devote their full time to their own family.

Furthermore, the mentality which honors women more for their work outside the home than for their work within the family must be overcome. This requires that men should truly esteem and love women with total respect for their personal dignity, and that society should create and develop conditions favoring work in the home.

— POPE JOHN PAUL II, *Familiaris Consortio*

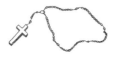

Dearest Lord, teach me to be generous: teach me to serve You as You deserve: to give and not count the cost, to fight and not to heed the wounds, to toil and not to seek for rest, to labor and not to ask for reward save that of knowing I am doing Your will.

— SAINT IGNATIUS LOYOLA

* * *

A thought, a prayer, a reflection...

NOVENA TO
SAINT GERARD MAJELLA 8

Dear Saint Gerard, you found a safe refuge and sure guide in every circumstance of your life in Mary the Mother of Jesus and our own Mother. Guide me, please, to a trusting and true devotion to Mary, and remind me often that the easiest way to union with Jesus is always to go to him through Mary.

Teach me also, Saint Gerard, the beauty and great value of the Rosary, that scriptural prayer that helps me to meditate on the main events in the life of Jesus and Mary. Amen.

SPIRITUAL COMMUNION

Dear Jesus, I believe with all of my heart
that you are truly and fully present in the Blessed Sacrament.
I wish I could be near you now.
Please forgive me all of my faults.
Since I cannot receive you sacramentally at this moment,
I pray that you will come into my soul spiritually. My heart
will embrace you as you fill me with your presence, Lord.
Thank you for your great love for me. Amen.

PRAYER TO OUR BLESSED MOTHER

Dear Blessed Mother Mary, my Queen and my Mother, continue to watch over me and stand beside me during the remaining weeks of my pregnancy. You have been so near throughout these past months. Please continue to help me and inspire me. Please keep me close to your son as only you can. Thank you for your tender loving care for my baby and me. Pray to Jesus for me, please, that I may receive the graces I most need to be a good and loving mother. Hail Mary, full of grace, the Lord is with thee, blessed art thou amongst women, and blessed is the fruit of thy womb, Jesus. Holy Mary, Mother of God, pray for us sinners, now and at the hour of our death. Amen.

PRAYER FOR A FAMILY

O dear Jesus, I confidently ask you to grant my family the graces that we need to serve you well. Please, dear Lord, protect and bless all of us who are present or away, living and deceased. Help us to hold tight to each other and know that prayer will unite our hearts and souls and keep us together. Amen.

A BLESSED MONTH

It won't be long now; you can almost count the days until the birth of your darling little one! It has been a heartfelt journey thus far, and surely you have grown spiritually as well as physically. Motherhood is a sublime privilege. Words cannot come close to expressing what you are experiencing as your child grows within you. Truly a mother knows. Your love for your child grows each day. Treasure and savor this beginning of your little one's life when he or she is thriving inside you, nourished by your life and love. These are special, holy times when your unborn baby is cradled and rocked in your womb. Even before your eyes meet each other, already you have been getting to know each other. Be at peace and be prayerful these last few weeks of pregnancy.

Enjoy these last few weeks. It is a fun and exciting time as you feather your nest, preparing for your baby's arrival.

Although you most likely have begun to feel uncomfortable because of your protruding abdomen, possible tummy upset, and lack of good sleep, remember that the day will soon be here when you are finally able to draw your precious little one close to your breast, to embrace, caress, and love your new child. Be sure to rest whenever you can. You need to reserve some strength for your delivery day! This will be a moment in your lifetime that you will never forget. It is an exhilarating, holy, tremendous time.

PRAYER FROM MY HEART

A prayer to my Lord from my heart in thanksgiving for this most beautiful gift of this new life within me:

Oh dear Lord _____

_____

_____

_____

_____

_____

_____

* * *

Reflections on My Eighth Month of Pregnancy

8

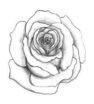

Your Ninth Month

"… but as for me and my house, we will serve the Lord."
— JOSHUA 24:15, RSV (CE)

Love is a fruit always in season, and no limit is set. Everyone can reach this love.
— BLESSED MOTHER TERESA OF CALCUTTA

*A*s the Second Vatican Council recalled, "Since parents have conferred life on their children, they have a most solemn obligation to educate their offspring. Hence, parents must be acknowledged as the first and foremost educators of their children. Their role as educators is so decisive that scarcely anything can compensate for their failure in it. For it devolves on parents to create a family atmosphere so animated with love and reverence for God and others that a well-rounded personal and social development will be fostered among the children. Hence, the family is the first school of those social virtues which every society needs."

— *Gravissimum Educationis*

WHAT'S HAPPENING WITH YOUR BABY?

During the ninth month, your baby's living quarters will become more cramped. Your baby will gain about two and a half pounds and grow about two inches this month.

Poor nourishment, poor health, and very hard work are some of the main causes of premature birth. Hence the absolute necessity for taking very good care of yourself while pregnant, especially during this ninth month. It is a good idea to stay as close to home as possible. Should you require medical help, you will be most comfortable with your own doctor and hospital. During the last trimester, your baby will receive gamma globulin from your blood, placenta, and amniotic fluid. It is thought that the gamma globulin helps to make the mother more immune to diseases during the last three months of pregnancy. Your baby will receive substances that will endow him with immunity to a wide variety of diseases. Your baby is pretty hardy by this ninth month because of the many immunities that are transferred from you. Your baby's protection from illness is good now but will be further improved by the antibodies in your breast milk, especially in colostrum, which is produced before your actual breast milk arrives. Even if you decide not to breast feed for long, giving your baby the awesome benefit of colostrum will get him or her off to a good start in life. Isn't God's design amazing? A mother's body is equipped with the perfect baby food, breast milk, providing the necessary nutrition at the right temperature. No need to heat it up or deal with bottles. No need for baby to be crying, wanting to eat while you are warming up formula. If possible, try to breastfeed your baby — it truly makes for a happy and healthy baby!

Your baby will most likely stop growing by the two hundred and sixtieth day, about a week before birth. God has seen to it that your baby has been preparing for birth by dropping and becoming engaged in the tight-fitting circle of pelvic bones. In most cases, a baby will remain there until birth.

PRAYER TO THE HOLY FAMILY

Lord Jesus Christ, you were raised by Mary and Joseph within the Holy Family in Nazareth. Your home was humble and holy. Help us discover the holiness in simplicity and obedience to our state of life. Help us to imitate the virtues of the Holy Family as we faithfully carry out our daily duties. Please also help us to find ways to seek out solitude even in the midst of our busy lives so that we may unite our hearts with yours, dear Jesus. Please, Blessed Mother Mary and good Saint Joseph, pray for our family and protect us. Amen.

ACT OF LOVE

O my God, You are all good and deserving of all my love. Therefore I love You, my Lord, above all things. I pray to love my neighbors as myself for the love of You. I ask forgiveness for all of my sins and the grace to always forgive others. Amen.

✻ ✻ ✻

A thought, a prayer, a reflection...

MOTHER'S DAILY PRAYER
FOR HER CHILDREN

O Mary, Immaculate Virgin, Mother of our Lord Jesus Christ, patroness of all mothers, I commend my beloved children to the Most Sacred Heart of your son, Jesus, and to your Immaculate Heart. Please assist our family and keep us always in your care. Please protect us from the snares of the devil and keep us on the road that leads to life. Help me to realize my sublime mission as a mother and help me be faithful to my duties for the good of my family and the good of the entire family of God.

Most Sacred Heart of Jesus, have mercy on us.
Immaculate Heart of Mary, pray for us.
My Guardian Angel, pray for me.
Holy Guardian Angel of our family, pray for us.
Saint Michael, pray for us.
Saint Joseph, husband of Mary, pray for us.
Saint Anne, mother of Mary, pray for us.
Saint Elizabeth, pray for us.
Saint Elizabeth Ann Seton, pray for us.
Saint Monica, pray for us.
Saint Augustine, pray for us.
Saint Gerard Majella, pray for us.
Blessed Mother Teresa of Calcutta, pray for us.
Amen.

or baptized persons, moreover, marriage invests the dignity of a sacramental sign of grace, inasmuch as it represents the union of Christ and of the Church.

Under this light, there clearly appear the characteristic marks and demands of conjugal love, and it is of supreme importance to have an exact idea of these.

This love is first of all fully human, that is to say, of the senses and the spirit at the same time. It is not, then, a simple transport of instinct and sentiment, but also, and principally, an act of the free will intended to endure and to grow by means of the joys and sorrows of daily life, in such a way that husband and wife become one heart and one only soul, and together attain their human perfection.

Again, this love is faithful and exclusive until death. Thus in fact do bride and groom conceive it to be on the day when they freely and in full awareness assume the duty of the marriage bond. A fidelity like this can sometimes be difficult, but is always possible, always noble and meritorious, as no one can deny. The example of so many married persons down through the centuries shows, not only that fidelity is according to the nature of marriage, but the communion between husband and wife, but also is destined to continue raising up new lives. "Marriage and conjugal love are by their nature ordained toward the begetting and education of children. Children are really the supreme gift of marriage and contribute very substantially to the welfare of their parents."

Hence, conjugal love requires in husband and wife an awareness of their mission of "responsible parenthood." Which today is rightly much insisted upon, and which also must be exactly understood. Consequently it is to be considered under different aspects which are legitimate and connected with one another.

— POPE PAUL VI, *Humanae Vitae*

NOVENA TO
SAINT ANNE 9

Saint Anne lived all of her life in the obscure town of Nazareth. She spent her days in a tiny house as a common person. Perhaps her ancestors lived in the royal palaces of David and his descendants. Anne, however, only knew of a common life, content in a cottage made beautiful by her love that filled it.

Once an unknown person, now thousands of churches and schools, hospitals and shrines have been built in Saint Anne's name throughout the generations. She now looks down from her mansion in Heaven, watching over the faithful and interceding for them in prayer.

PRAYER TO SAINT ANNE

Dear Saint Anne, patroness of mothers, please listen to my humble prayers to you. I ask you to continue to guide me throughout this month when my baby is growing within me. Pray to the Heavenly Father, please, to grant me the graces I most need so that I will mother my child with a pure love all the devotion of my heart. Help me to always hold onto hope as you have done. Guide me, please, to look for quiet moments to seek our Lord so that I will use this pregnancy wisely to be open to God's love for me and my baby in a special way. Help me to come closer to your daughter, Mary, as I pray throughout this pregnancy. Amen.

A MOTHER'S PRAYER
TO THE SACRED HEART

O Sacred Heart of Jesus, I present to you this day the dearest treasure I possess, which resides in my being — my unborn baby. Thank you for the great gift of motherhood. Please bless my innocent child now and forever. Please grant my baby the graces of sobriety, wisdom, knowledge, piety, and a holy love for you so that my child will grow up in the graces of your holy Commandments. Please preserve him or her from all danger, spiritual and physical. Defend my baby with your powerful protection. Please take my baby into the sanctuary of your tender and sacred heart to remain safe and blessed all the days of his or her life and one day with you in eternity. Amen.

Because we cannot see Christ, we cannot express our love to Him in person. But our neighbor we can see, and we can do for him or her what we would love to do for Jesus if He were visible.

Let us be open to God so that He can use us. Let us put love into our actions, beginning in the family, in the neighborhood, in the street. It is difficult, but there is where the work begins. We are the co-workers of Christ, a fruit bearing branch of the vine.

— BLESSED MOTHER TERESA OF CALCUTTA

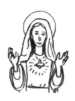

PRAYER TO JESUS

Dear Jesus, I thank you for the amazing gift of my unborn baby who awaits birth along with me. Help me to see with my heart and mind that I stand in your place before my children. I have an incredible responsibility to raise my children in the truth of their faith. Grant me the grace to be faithful to my calling as a mother to innocent children, created in your image, who depend on me for direction in life. Help me to be open to your will at all times, even when difficult, knowing you will give me strength and grace for the asking. Help me to put love into all my actions with my family, knowing that when I am serving my family, I am also serving you, dear Lord. Amen.

The modern Christian family is often tempted to be discouraged and distressed at the growth of its difficulties; it is an eminent form of love to give it back its reasons for confidence in itself, in the riches that it possesses by nature and grace, and in the mission that God has entrusted to it. Yes indeed, the families of today must be called back to their original position. They must follow Christ.

— POPE JOHN PAUL II, *Familiaris Consortio*

Mothers are the heart of the home; they build family life by wanting, loving, and taking care of their children. Mothers make the home a center of love. Their role is sometimes hard, but there is the example of the Blessed Virgin, who teaches us to be good with our children.

— BLESSED MOTHER TERESA OF CALCUTTA

MOTHER OF BODY AND SOUL

The Fiat of the Annunciation is repeated every time a woman accepts the incarnation of love. Every mother, when she responds to the Lord with her generous "yes" to new life, accepts motherhood of a new human being's body and soul. The Creator's majesty descends upon her marriage as she becomes the guardian of this new precious life. Motherhood remains an awesome privilege.

* * *

A thought, a prayer, a reflection...

THE GLORIOUS MYSTERIES
OF THE ROSARY
(See above pages 67–71)

I. The Resurrection

II. The Ascension

III. The Descent of the Holy Spirit

IV. The Assumption

V. The Coronation

PRAYER TO SAINT JOSEPH

O dear Saint Joseph, Saint Teresa of Avila was forever singing your praises. She taught us that we should turn to you in all necessities and that you will help. As head of the Holy Family, you certainly knew what responsibility was all about. You underwent trials of poverty, persecution, and exile and glorified God as you defended and protected Jesus and the Blessed Mother, always keeping them safe. Please ask our dear Lord to look kindly on me, an expectant mother. I wish to raise my child in a holy home. Please pray that I will receive the graces I most need to accomplish this awesome task. Please also pray for my husband that he will be inspired to imitate your great virtues. Amen.

Among the fundamental tasks of the Christian family is its ecclesial task: the family is placed at the service of the building up of the Kingdom of God in history by participating in the life and mission of the Church.

— POPE JOHN PAUL II, *Familiaris Consortio*

THE HEART OF THE DEEPEST TRUTH

Pope John Paul II told us in "The Role of the Christian Family in the Modern World" (*Familiaris Consortio*) that "the Church knows the path by which the family can reach the heart of the deepest truth about itself. The Church has learned this path at the school of Christ and the school of history interpreted in the light of the Spirit. She does not impose, it but she feels an urgent need to propose it to everyone without fear and indeed with great confidence and hope, although she knows that the Good News included the subject of the Cross. But it is through the Cross that the family can attain the fullness of its being and the perfection of its love."

Dear Lord, help families all over the world to raise their children in love, seeking the truth above all else by following Christ. Grant us the graces to remain a prayerful family, creating a domestic church within our home, remaining faithful to our day-to-day duties, bearing with each other and life's tribulations. Help us to remember that love begins at home and that we should be attentive to one another's needs. We pray to be always open and generous to the needs of our neighbor, as well, joyfully giving of ourselves, helping to fulfill God's will while living out the Gospel.

Help us to seek first the kingdom of God, knowing in our hearts that it will not always be easy, but our reward will be great in Heaven and even upon Earth as we strive to reach the perfection and fullness of God's love in the blessedness of our family.

Jesus said that we are much more important in the eyes of His Father than the grass, the birds, and the flowers of the earth. And that if He takes care of these things, how much more He would take care of His own life in us. He cannot deceive us. Life is God's greatest gift to human beings, and humans are created in the image of God. Life belongs to God and we do not have the right to destroy it.

— BLESSED MOTHER TERESA OF CALCUTTA

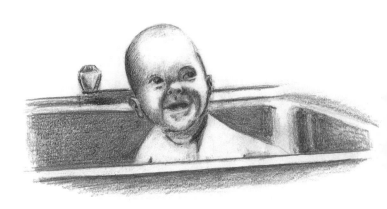

NOVENA TO
SAINT GERARD MAJELLA 9

Dear Saint Gerard Majella, I trust in your powerful intercession before the Blessed Trinity. I present my request to you now as I am carrying my baby. Please also pray for the graces I need to be the mother I should be. Please pray that God will instill within my heart the same love that you had for God's holy will. Please guide me and watch over my baby and me. Amen.

SPIRITUAL COMMUNION

Dear Jesus, I believe with all of my heart
that you are truly and fully present in the Blessed Sacrament.
I wish I could be near you now.
Please forgive me of all my faults.
Since I cannot receive you sacramentally at this moment,
I pray that you will come into my soul spiritually. My heart will
    embrace you as you fill me with your presence, Lord.
Thank you for your great love for me.
Amen.

PRAYER TO OUR BLESSED MOTHER

Dear Blessed Mother Mary, my Mother in Heaven, thank you for remaining by my side during my pregnancy. Thank you for the graces that I received because of your prayers to your son for me. I ask for your help especially now when I am soon to give birth. Pray for me, please, that I will have the necessary strength and that my unborn baby may enter this world safely. I ask that you will continue to show me how I am to be a virtuous mother.

Help me to be at peace while I care for and love this little child of God. Protect our family, and please always inspire my husband and me to work together for the good of our family and for God's glory. Whatever suffering we may have to endure, please keep us together in Christ's love. Please remind us to find time for prayer, alone and together, seeking strength and guidance so that we may raise our family in a manner that is pleasing to God. Hail Mary, full of grace, the Lord is with thee, blessed art thou amongst women, and blessed is the fruit of thy womb, Jesus. Holy Mary, Mother of God, pray for us sinners, now and at the hour of our death. Amen.

A GRACE-FILLED MONTH

You are reaching the end of this God-given journey, during which your life and love nourished your unborn child. It is a glorious time of joyful expectation awaiting your baby's birth. Savor the memories of your little one's beginnings. Thank God for the gift of this child and for the gift of these past nine months of prayer and preparation for the new journey on which you will soon embark — the most noble vocation of motherhood. Oh the joys that await you when you meet this little person, who is flesh of your flesh, who has been kicking you from inside your womb, who has already been listening to your voice, whom you have rocked with your every move. Soon you will be able to hold your sweet baby and cradle him or her in your arms at last, pouring your motherly love upon him. You and your husband will experience true joy and sweet happiness. Get as much rest as you can so you are strong for childbirth and regain your strength before too long.

God bless you and your child, your husband, and your family, now and forever.

Do not search for Jesus in faroff lands; He is not there. He is in you. Just keep the lamp burning and you will always see Him.

Jesus has chosen each and every one of you to be His love and His light in the world.

— BLESSED TERESA OF CALCUTTA

PRAYER FROM MY HEART

A prayer to my Lord from my heart in thanksgiving for this most beautiful gift of this new life within me:

Oh dear Lord _____

_____

_____

_____

_____

_____

_____

* * *

Reflections on My Ninth Month of Pregnancy

*F*or every believer, and especially for Christian families, the humble dwelling place in Nazareth is an authentic school of the Gospel. Here we admire, put into practice, the divine plan to make the family an intimate community of life and love; here we learn that every Christian family is called to be a small domestic church that must shine with the Gospel virtues. Recollection and prayer, mutual understanding and respect, personal discipline and community, asceticism and a spirit of sacrifice, work and solidarity are typical features that make the family of Nazareth a model for every home.

— POPE JOHN PAUL II, December 30, 2001

* * *

Reflections on My Pregnancy

* * *

Reflections on My Pregnancy

✳ ✳ ✳

Choices of Names for My Baby

BECOME WHAT WE ARE

The family finds in the plan of God the Creator and Redeemer not only its *identity*, what it is, but also its *mission*, what it can and should *do*. The role that God calls the family to perform in history derives from what the family is; its role represents the dynamic and existential development of what it is. Each family finds within itself a summons that cannot be ignored, and that specifies both its dignity and its responsibility: family, *become* what you *are*.

— POPE JOHN PAUL II, *Familiaris Consortio*

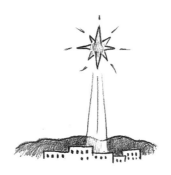

* * *

Hopes for my baby:

* * *

Hopes for my baby:

PRAYER OF BLESSING FOR MY NEWBORN BABY

O Dear God _____

_____

_____

_____

_____

_____

_____

_____

_____

_____

_____

_____

_____

_____

_____

_____

_____

_____

_____

_____

_____

A Word from the Author

I wrote this book while I was on complete bed rest because of serious complications during a pregnancy with my fifth child, Mary-Catherine. I had four other active children in the household at that time, and I think our good Lord literally had to make me remain still in order to give me the opportunity to get these words on paper that can now be shared with other mothers. I felt inspired to write what was in my heart, to share the graces and blessings of my pregnancies and motherhood with other expectant mothers.

As a mother raising five children, I am very familiar with what a mother these days is up against. I find it is important to encourage other mothers in any way that I can. Women today live with a barrage of mixed messages directed at them, which may cause them to feel confused about their roles in their families and in the world. We live in a time when our society pushes women to pursue careers outside the home and tells them not to be satisfied with the sublime vocation of motherhood. We are told that our worth is measured by the size of our paycheck. Mothers are advised that motherhood is "just" changing diapers, doing laundry, and performing other mundane, mindless, or unimportant tasks. However, we know that the tasks we do as mothers are the acts of love that keep our families together in intimate communion and at peace. God uses these loving acts as a means of sanctifying our families.

I firmly believe that our children are our most precious treasures and that they need and deserve our unconditional love, guidance, and presence. Although I know that the bills pile up mercilessly and it may be difficult to make ends meet at times, being present to our little ones is one of our most crucial duties as mothers and should be first and foremost in our minds when deciding whether or not to work outside the home, and if so, when it would be most appropriate. A mother's love and devotion and presence are indispensable components in a baby's life. We should delay working outside the home if possible in order to have the time and energy we need to mother our young children properly. This is an important issue to ponder during our pregnancies so we will be prepared to plan our lives accordingly.

For some mothers, it may seem easier or more satisfying to go out into the world and get a pat on the back and praise from coworkers or employers than to go without praise at times for a job well done in the home. We need to remind ourselves that, in the tapestry of motherhood, the many sacrifices that are necessary in our commitment and devotion to our children are interwoven with the wonderful rewards of raising them. Sometimes these sacrifices may mean giving up or putting aside other worthwhile pursuits so we may devote our full attention to our children and our family.

It is unlikely that a mother's work in the home will ever make the headlines. But the extraordinary love that a mother puts into her ordinary routine makes her role become worthwhile and quite astonishing! Let us pray that this amazing role will be recognized for its intrinsic irreplaceable value and the creating hand of God within it.

Acknowledgments

FOR ALL OF THE MOTHERS IN MY LIFE:

To my mother, Alexandra Mary Uzwiak Cooper, in loving memory and gratitude for bringing me into this world against doctor's orders and raising me with her tender love and grace in our large family. She taught me the necessity of prayer and how to give without ever counting the cost.

In loving memory and gratitude to my grandmother Alexandra Theresa Karasiewicz Uzwiak for her inexhaustible love, guidance, and inspiration. Her smile, her laugh, and her lessons of love and prayer live on in my life.

To my godmother, Aunt Bertha Uzwiak Barosky, in gratitude for her loving prayers and guidance throughout my life, which she continues in her sweet optimistic way to bestow upon me even now.

In loving memory of Blessed Teresa of Calcutta, my gratitude for her cherished lessons of love and holy living that have deeply inspired me. Her consistent encouragement to me to continue to write to help others has certainly given me much courage and motivation. I thank her for her poignant and tender words that form the foreword of this book and quotes throughout. Her faith in me and love for me has left a permanent imprint on my heart.

To dear Mother Mary, our Blessed Mother, who has always watched over me during my lifetime, my gratitude for her motherly influence, love, and protection that has forever been my saving grace.

TO ALL OTHERS I HOLD DEAR:

With a special loving thanks to my daughter Chaldea for her beautiful illustrations of my children as babies and of myself that help to enhance the message of this book.

In loving memory of my father, Eugene Joseph Cooper, who along with my mother brought me into this world, my gratitude for his love and support, working hard to care for our large family.

To my brothers and sisters — Alice Jean, Gene, Gary, Barbara, Tim, Michael, and David. Thank you for all the great times throughout the years. Thank you for loving me.

To my very dear friend and spiritual guide, Father Bill C. Smith, thank you for your cherished friendship, love, and guidance. Your amazing guidance has certainly helped to mold me into who I am. I will forever be thankful.

To my husband, David, my partner and best friend, thank you for believing in me and loving me. You are the wind beneath my wings.

In loving memory of an amazing and saintly person of our time, dear Pope John Paul the Great, my gratitude for his inexhaustible wisdom and blessings in the profound and selfless love of his shepherding, which I was able to benefit from throughout a good part of my lifetime.

Additionally, I thank you, dear Lord Jesus, for putting me still and on complete bed rest during my precarious pregnancy, inspiring and enabling me to write down my thoughts, prayers, and reflections on pregnancy and motherhood so these words may be shared with other mothers on the pilgrimage of mother-hood. Thank you, dear Lord, for your love!

I would also like to thank Roy M. Carlisle, John Jones, Michael Egan and Gwendolin Herder at The Crossroad Publishing Company for having faith in me to go forward with this book. It was very providential to meet Roy and John on the Feast of the Immaculate Heart of Mary at the Book Expo in New York and to be given the opportunity and privilege to talk with them about my work. I thank them for being a very important part of this book coming to fruition. I would like to thank Nancy Neal and Linabel Herrera also from The Crossroad Publishing Company for their help, especially for their thoughtful attention to the decorative details of this book. It has been a great pleasure and honor to work with all of the team.

About the Author

Donna-Marie Cooper O'Boyle speaks to a mother's heart about the blessings, grace, and lessons she learned throughout her spiritual journey during motherhood. She has received awards for her work and is the author of two previous books.

Embracing family life, she became a mother of five. She also served as a prioress and a mistress of novices for the Third Order of Saint Dominic branch that she helped to start, founded a branch of the Lay Missionaries of Charity, taught religious education for over twenty years, and was a eucharistic minister to 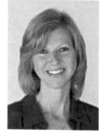 the sick. She founded the Angels of Mercy, the Marian Mothers, Apostles of the Blessed Sacrament, and friends of Veronica, an outreach program for senior citizens and the lonely. She is a Lay Missionary of Charity.

In God's divine providence, Donna-Marie met Blessed Teresa of Calcutta and remained in contact with her for a decade, during which they met and corresponded. Donna-Marie is passionate about sharing her inspiration and the heart-to-hearts she had with her beloved friend, Blessed Teresa of Calcutta, with other mothers, to encourage them and help them to see the sublimity of their vocation. Donna-Marie lectures on topics relationg to Catholic women and can be reached at her website www.donnacooperoboyle.com. She also posts daily updates to her blog at www.donnamariecooperoboyle.com.

The Heart of Motherhood:
Finding Holiness in the Catholic Home
Donna-Marie Cooper O'Boyle
ISBN 0-8245-2403-9
Paperback

When dirty dishes and laundry start to pile up, it's easy for Catholic mothers to believe that the call to sanctity is for someone else. But we are all called to holiness, and mothers have their own unique calling. In *The Heart of Motherhood*, Donna-Marie draws from her own life as a mother to five children, and from the teachings of Mother Teresa on home, family life, and prayer. With guidance for a deeper prayer life amid the chaos, we learn that our entire lives as mothers can become a prayer. With anecdotes, devotions, original prayers, helpful tips, and inspiration for achieving loving communication with God, this book helps mothers keep their sanity intact while seeking the sanctity to which everyone is called.

Modern Mothering:
How to Teach Kids to Say What They Feel
and Feel What They Way
Tian Dayton
ISBN 0-8245-2340-7
Paperback

In this tender and wise little book, Dr. Tian Dayton discusses the latest techniques for nourishing sound emotinal development in our children while exploring opportunities for spiritual growth in motherhood. By weaving together everyday experiences and easy to understand explanations of scientific research, she hilights the importance of personal authenticity. Children become strong and develop confidence when they can say what they feel and feel what they say and we become stronger and more confident as we model emotional, intellectual, and spiritual health. For more information, visit www.modernmothering.com.

Tian Dayton, Ph.D. is a psychologist and creative arts therapist in private practice in New York City. She holds an M.A. in educational psychology and is a certified Montessori teacher. Dr. Dayton is the author of fourteen books and a frequent guest expert on TV and radio. She lives with her husband, Brandt and near her two children Marina and Alex.

Kristi: So Thin the Veil
Peter Beaulieu
ISBN 0-8245-2398-9
Paperback

A husband's devotion to his wife, and his wife's devotion to God in the midst of cancer and physical suffering, shine through on every page of this remarkable book. Kristi is the tale of one woman of unshakable faith and courage, and a testimony to the power of women of faith everywhere. In Kristi's life we see, as through a veil, glimpses of the light of heaven. "Beautifully written, this book is a riveting and inspiring story of faith, a provocative reflection on death and eternal life, and a love poem."

—Dale Ahlquist, President, American Chesterton Society

Check your local bookstore for availability.
To order directly from the publisher,
please call 1-800-707-0670 for Customer Service
or visit our Web site at www.cpcbooks.com.
For catalog orders, please send your request to the address below.
THE CROSSROAD PUBLISHING COMPANY
16 Penn Plaza, Suite 1550, New York, NY 10001
All prices subject to change.